Homelessness and Mental Illness

This book explores the trajectories of social suffering, exclusion, and victimisation of homeless persons with mental illness in India. It uses a Critical Ethnographic approach to study their lived experiences associated with downward mobilisation and the challenges in the process of recovery and empowerment.

Using theoretical and methodological implications, the volume highlights the experiences of this marginalised population through their voices instead of relying on epidemiological data only. It presents stories that show how such persons celebrate their abilities to tolerate all forms of ostracisation and endure their sufferings with fortitude. This book discusses how "hope," as a part of their experience, catalyses the process of recovery and empowerment and helps them develop meaningful social ties to access valued social resources. It further brings to light the difficulties experienced by service providers in providing service due to a lack of resources and support at a systemic level and awareness about mental illness among various stakeholders.

This book will be of interest to students, teachers, and researchers of social psychology, clinical psychology, community psychology, and sociology. It will also be helpful for academicians, policymakers, social workers, mental health practitioners, and NGO personnel.

Prama Bhattacharya is an Assistant Professor of Psychology School of Humanities, Social Sciences and Management, Indian Institute of Technology Bhubaneswar, Odisha, India.

Homelessness is related to various psychiatric disorders and often it is not clear what comes first. Increasing our understanding through review and research Dr Bhattacharya comes up with some innovative ideas. The book will be of major interest to clinicians and NGOs but, more importantly, to policymakers. Looking after vulnerable individuals is the first task of any society, and this book contributes in a major way to that debate and discussion.

Dinesh Bhugra, *Professor Emeritus, Mental Health &*
Cultural Diversity, Institute of Psychiatry, Psychology &
Neuroscience, Kings College, London

Bhattacharya's work deep dives into complex problems around homelessness and mental illness. Lived experience contributes to diverse narratives, textured and layered with unique insights. The author has attempted to straddle multiple social worlds that contribute to the social imagination around "madness" and being "homed" or "homeless." Limited scholarly work in this field has emerged from the Global South, and I congratulate her for taking the lead on this front.

Vandana Gopikumar, *Co-Founder, The Banyan &*
The Banyan Academy of Leadership in Mental Health (BALM)

The journey of mind champions from despair to hope is put forth by Dr Bhattacharya in *Homelessness and Mental Illness: Exploring the Lived Experience in India* in a compelling style which does not allow us to invisibilise the homeless persons with psychosocial disability on the streets anymore.

Sarbani Das Roy, *Co-Founder and Secretary, Iswar Sankalpa*

Homelessness and Mental Illness
Exploring the Lived Experience in India

Prama Bhattacharya

Routledge
Taylor & Francis Group

LONDON AND NEW YORK

First published 2024
by Routledge
4 Park Square, Milton Park, Abingdon, Oxon OX14 4RN

and by Routledge
605 Third Avenue, New York, NY 10158

Routledge is an imprint of the Taylor & Francis Group, an informa business

British Library Cataloguing-in-Publication Data
A catalogue record for this book is available from the British Library

ISBN: 978-1-032-19572-8 (hbk)
ISBN: 978-1-032-66206-0 (pbk)
ISBN: 978-1-032-66205-3 (ebk)

DOI: 10.4324/9781032662053

Typeset in Sabon
by SPi Technologies India Pvt Ltd (Straive)

My Parents and My Brother

Contents

Figures

Foreword

The socio-economic differentials have a long civilisational history. Against this backdrop, it is remarkable that in the Indian ethos, the poor, vulnerable, and destitute called *Daridra Narayana* have been traditionally given an important place, and in an individual capacity, a Grihastha or householder had a debt called *Bhuta Rina* which demanded fulfilling obligations to take care of the needy persons. The current wave of socio-economic changes, however, has brought in destabilising changes and has been posing an enormous challenge for the people on the margins of society. As a result, the needs for food and shelter continue to be a major item on the agenda of social development of the government. Over the years the processes of globalisation, urbanisation, and the attendant ideology of consumerism and individualism are leading to transformation in the social ecology. As a result, the shrinking of the socially shared public resources and weakening of community support are resulting in the dwindling of provisions.

Indeed, the necessary structures for underprivileged people have been waning, and the incidence of homelessness has evinced a considerable rise in the number of homeless people in the urban sector of the Indian population. This is often accompanied by physical and mental health issues of various kinds. The homeless people are multiply disadvantaged, and their quality of life gets substantially compromised. The conditions of civic amenities available to them are quite varied across different sections of the population and in the different regions of India. Within the broad category of homeless people, those with severe mental illnesses (HMI) happen to constitute one of the most vulnerable segments of society. It is, therefore, gratifying to see the move on the part of social scientists who have a tendency to be preoccupied with the description of normal and ordinary lives. In doing so, Dr Prama Bhattacharya has extended the boundaries of the discipline by challenging the individual-centric, universalistic, and psychopathology-oriented focus.

However, the study of HMIs falls at the intersection of several disciplines. The present author is critical of the disability lens adopted in earlier research. The alternative view advanced by her considers capturing the strengths and resilience among these people and fostering these psychological assets to cope with the challenges. With a view to enable HMIs to survive in hostile environments, a framework consisting of social suffering, recovery, and empowerment is advanced. The empirical work reported in volume is refreshing. It documents and reports the results of an empirical inquiry into the lives of a group of rehabilitated HMI persons and their service providers. The study was undertaken with the help of semi-structured interviews and participant observation in two metro cities. The developmental trajectories documented in the life narratives of ex-HMIs offer an engaging account of the emerging patterns. The experiences of service providers highlight the process of recovery and empowerment in HMI persons and offer insights into the rehabilitation of HMIs. It is rightly observed that when homelessness co-occurs with severe mental illness, the lack of resources makes it more difficult for HMIs to exit the vicious cycle. The volume has also situated the problem in the global context and in the relevant disciplinary matrix. The framework of social suffering, recovery, and empowerment envisaged by the present researcher is convincing.

Dr Bhattacharya has traced the diverse developmental trajectories found in the lives of HMIs. The life stories presented are of those ex-HMI category persons who could garner hope as a way of life through their relationships with significant others. These self-reflections on their experiential journeys contributing towards recovery and empowerment illustrate the ways these people dealt with the hurdles of a multitude of social suffering. The volume also provides accounts of the experience of service providers and draws attention to the factors that have motivated them and the challenges encountered while implementing rehabilitation programmes.

This work signifies a departure from the dominant trend in social science research. By capturing, articulating, and sharing the reality of the homeless as experienced by the participants themselves. Using empathy and giving space and opportunity to voice their views changes has made the appreciation of the phenomenon of homelessness more realistic. I congratulate Dr Bhattacharya for undertaking this innovative work and bringing the problem of homelessness to the centre stage of social scientific discourse. I hope that she will maintain this spirit and continue to enrich the discipline.

Girishwar Misra
Former Vice Chancellor, Mahatma Gandhi Antarrashtriya Hindi
Vishvavidyalaya, Wardha, and Former Head of the Department of
Psychology, University of Delhi, Delhi

Acknowledgements

After laboriously scrawling a staggering 60,000 words for this volume, I found myself in a pickle when it came to penning the *Acknowledgement*. It's given that the leitmotif of an acknowledgement section will exude a pervasive aura of gratitude. The pressing issue, however, at hand is who do I not acknowledge! Expressing gratitude to chosen few is quite the undertaking. *Thus, I shall bestow monikers upon those scant entities, bereft of whom I would not have rendered this celestial orb, professionally and personally. Here it goes...*

My eternal gratitude is owed to my participants, who graciously entrusted me with the privilege of delving into the depths of their existence, baring their souls with a vulnerability that belied the anguish that accompanied those recollections. I've always wished to utilise my book as a platform to amplify those voices tragically overlooked and unheard by the stakeholders. I sincerely hope that this volume fulfils its intended purpose, whatever that may be.

I must express my deepest appreciation to the entire *Iswar Sankalpa* and *The Banyan* crew for their steadfast assistance.

Thank you, *Prof. Kumar Ravi Priya*, for your unwavering belief in my amorphous musings, for giving them a structure and making them a reality. You are that mentor and philosopher guide any scholar would be lucky to have. This book is as much your dream as it is mine.

I am ever indebted *to my teachers at the Department of Humanities and Social Sciences, IIT Kanpur – Professors A.K. Sinha and Vineet Sahoo and at Kolkata – Professors Leena Nair Sengupta, Deepsikha Ray, and Atanu Kumar Dogra.*

My long-suffering friends – *Madhurima, Parama, Priya, Pourabi, and Nidhi* – I love you for being by me even through my long tenures of silence and for not judging me, ever! I wish I could acknowledge this more often!

Thank you, Debanjan, for your unconditional support.

Bhai, my partner in crimes – Thank you for everything you do for me and make me do for you, for your blind faith in me and your un(?)conditional love!

Maa-Baba, you nurture my dreams like they are yours! Your thirst for knowledge is contagious. You taught me to work hard, stay true to my philosophy, and be kind and humble. Your monumental support in all things I do is too immense to pen down! I am grateful!

Prama Bhattacharya
IIT Bhubaneswar, Odisha

1 Homeless Individuals with Serious Mental Illnesses

Global and Indian Scenario

A Beautiful Mind Revisited!

She was sitting and weaving a colourful basket on her dorm bed the first time I saw her. A woman in her mid-twenties, modestly dressed, almost in a meditative posture. It was at the shelter house for homeless women with psycho-social disabilities run by a non-governmental organisation (NGO) called The Banyan. "I will tell you my story if you listen," she replied as I approached her for an interview.

> I do not remember my mother. She died when I was two. Soon after, my father left me with a couple who were his relatives to take care of me. He died when I was seven. This couple had two daughters of their own, both older to me. I always knew they were not my parents and was reminded by them that they were doing me a favour a by letting me stay with them. I was often beaten badly by the mother. There was always discrimination between their daughters and me. I was sent to school but also made to do household chores like washing dishes and clothes. The two sisters, they would also criticise me.
>
> When I had just completed high school, their mother died. They became more aggressive towards me after that. I became outraged and frustrated. I came out of the house after finding a job as a caretaker in an orphanage. I started living there. It was during this time that my mental health started deteriorating. I could hear voices talking to me, and I would not eat or bathe for days. The orphanage doctor sent me to a psychiatrist, and treatment started. My colleagues reached out to my foster family. The sisters came and took me home. They took away all my money, whatever I had earned. My medicines also got discontinued.
>
> I ran away from their home one day. I do not know why, but I came to the station and boarded a train. I did not know where I was going. I had nothing with me. A few men attacked and raped me on the train, and I could do nothing. This train was going to someplace in Gujrat. The police rescued me from the platform in very poor condition and

DOI: 10.4324/9781032662053-1

took me to an NGO. I was treated with medicines there. I stayed there for almost two months. They then contacted The Banyan, and I was brought back here. This was three years ago.

Prathiva confided to Dr VG, the co-founder of The Banyan, which gave her life a new direction,

I told her how I lose control over myself and give up when they (voices) instruct me. Then, she asked me to join a college diploma course in Community Psychology. I had already studied up to class 12. So, I entered college and finished that course.

Her decision to join the diploma course initiated the recovery process and gave her a new purpose in life

I learned how to seek out people with mental illnesses in the community, help elders who are thrown out of their homes, and provide treatment for the mentally ill in the city. I helped four individuals get their disability certificates. I brought five people from the community to The Banyan.

Prathiva acknowledges the guidance and services received from The Banyan. She wants to pursue a career in Community Mental Health with Dr VG's guidance, whom she considers her guardian, her "new" family.

Prathiva reminded me of John Nash when she revealed her strategy to deal with her auditory hallucinations, "I can do multiple tasks at a time. We do listen to music and do some other work simultaneously. Similarly, I would have voices instead of music playing in the background and do my studies. I can do that." Her insight into her mental health condition and the challenges awaiting her became critical in her relentless struggle against the odds. "My illness is a hindrance. But it would not be a hindrance if I keep taking my medicines. I can overcome it if it is under control," she reflects.

Prathiva received the resources to venture into a realistic process for her recovery and empowerment. However, she required the right amount of support from the community and the stakeholders to make those resources accessible to her. The Banyan became that support to her. This book attempts to provide space for the journeys of many such voices whose stories have remained unheard and invisible to society.

Homelessness and Serious Mental Illnesses within the Global and Indian Context

I have grown up in one of the largest cosmopolitan metro cities of India, Kolkata. Because of her innate charms, this city always seems full of light and life. However, beneath that, there is a city of chaos and clamour where these invisible people exist. They have been all around the city, at every other street corner. I would often come across them in my everyday life. Every time, the very sight would send a shiver down my spine. I instinctively questioned, "Who are they? From where do they come? How did they end up being on the streets? Who cares for them? How do they survive these inordinately hostile environments? What would happen to them next?" Intending to seek the answers, I had no direction on how to pursue them.

During this time, I came across a newspaper article (Bandyopadhyay, 2014) in one of the leading dailies of my city. It was on homeless people who have a serious mental illness (SMI), the state's apathy towards them, and how a non-profit organisation had been trying to provide community-based rehabilitation to this population despite all odds to make them once again visible to society. Coming across that article, I finally found that direction. I chose to indulge myself in the quest to get those answers through my doctoral research project by studying their lived experiences and exploring their life stories. I thought that pursuing these questions would enable me to create space for their voice towards a life with human dignity.

The following few pages will provide a brief understanding of the concepts of homelessness and SMIs in the global context with an emphasis on India. To situate homelessness, it becomes relevant to understand the idea of home, mainly because its meaning has varied across disciplines. Following a discussion on home and homelessness in the global and Indian context, I would discuss the antecedents and consequences of homelessness that would help to establish SMI as both and the vicious loop it creates for homeless individuals suffering from SMI. Lastly, I would consider the statistics of homeless people with serious mental illness (HMI) in India to contextualise the severity of the phenomenon in India.

What Is Home?

When I started writing this chapter and more explicitly answering the question of whom we call homeless, I was intrigued by the fact that I was not sure what home meant for me! So, I asked a few colleagues – "What is home for you?" While one answered – "Where I can be myself unflinchingly," another responded, "Warmth, understanding of small things, unconditional love and support. My little nest with a non-judgemental atmosphere." To my brother, who left home at 18, home is that space where he had shared his childhood with me, and now, it is that niche in his dormitory where he can do all the things he loves without any external interference. To a colleague trying to understand the imaginary conception of homeland in diaspora literature, home is a space where she can find physical and mental comfort. The Concise Oxford Dictionary (1999) defined home as "the place where one lives permanently." The resonating themes in all these understandings of the home being – space, autonomy, love and belongingness, and security. In the arena of academic understanding, home is a multidimensional concept, an ideology that is shaped by the lived experience of a person.

Defining Homelessness: The International Perspective

The United Nations (UN)-Habitat Report of 2015 declared that there is no internationally agreed definition of homelessness (2015). Depending on the socio-economic, socio-political, and socio-cultural context, the definition varies. The definition that the UN proposes for statistical purposes considers homeless households as follows:

> ...households without a shelter that would fall within the scope of living quarters. They carry their few possessions with them, sleeping in the streets, in doorways or on piers, or in any other space, on a more or less random basis.
>
> (UN, 1998, p. 50)

Because of the accommodation orientation of the above definition and classification, commentators on homelessness often argued against the use of the term and for replacing it with houselessness or rooflessness as they fail to do justice to the dynamics of the concept of home or the lack of it. They are also not sufficient to portray the reality of homelessness in every country. However, when it comes to defining homelessness, Tipple and Speak (2009) posed that:

> ... home is qualitatively different from adequate shelter in that it provides a set of essential social and emotional requirements separate from shelter and which cannot be provided by adequate shelter alone.
>
> (p. 4)

Therefore, a shelter might not be considered enough or holistic until it meets those social and emotional requirements.

Though the initial conceptualisation of homelessness has been based mainly on research on industrialised developed nations, the context of homelessness is much different in developing countries. However, a working definition of homelessness would be required for any nation for intervention or policy development because how we define homelessness would determine how we count them.

The Indian Perspective of Homelessness

At par with the accommodation-oriented definition, Tipple and Speak (2005) cited that the Census of India (2001) uses the term houseless households. In the census, households are conceptualised as individuals who stay together and share the kitchen. Houseless households or homeless people have been conceptualised by the Census of India (2011) as "the persons who are not living in Census houses, with possible places of habitat including pavements, roadsides, at railway platforms, under staircases, inside drainage pipes, at temple-mandaps, or in the open" (as cited in Goel et al., 2017, p. 88). A census house is a structure with a roof. This definition fails to include those living in institutions (except for shelter houses meant specifically for the homeless) or those sharing the accommodation involuntarily (Tipple & Speak, 2005). While it might be appropriate as a working definition for land or housing policies and the census, it fails to capture the complexity and multidimensionality of home and the lack of it. On the contrary, few working definitions used by NGOs are more holistic, broad, and inclusive. For example, Aashray Adhikar Abhiyan (AAA) defines home and homeless as follows:

> [one] who has no place to call a home in the city. By home is meant a place which not only provides a shelter but takes care of one's health, social, cultural and economic needs. Home offers a holistic care and security (sic).
>
> (as cited in Tipple & Speak, 2005, p. 347)

To operationalise the definition of homelessness in this book, I would consider this definition as provided by AAA. This definition has moved beyond the accommodation orientation of the earlier descriptions. It includes those essential social and emotional factors that make a shelter adequate to become a home.

Factors Contributing to Homelessness in India

The previous section has already established that homelessness is not merely a lack of a "structure with a roof." Therefore, to trace the pathway that leads people to homelessness, one must move beyond the most apparent reason for homelessness, that is, lack of affordable housing and delve into the other factors that trace the pathway to homelessness (Figure 1.1).

Understanding the contribution of homelessness is difficult because the factors that explain contemporary homelessness are complex, intertwined, and ambiguous. The ambiguity in the concept of causes stems from the factor that they vary across a wide array of dimensions from distal to proximal, on the one hand, to predisposing to precipitating reasons or individual cases of homelessness against aggregate homelessness.

Socio-economic Factors:

- Among the factors contributing to homelessness in India, *poverty* has been identified to be the most influential since it makes the availability of all other resources difficult (Gopikumar, Narasimhan et al., 2015, p. 43).

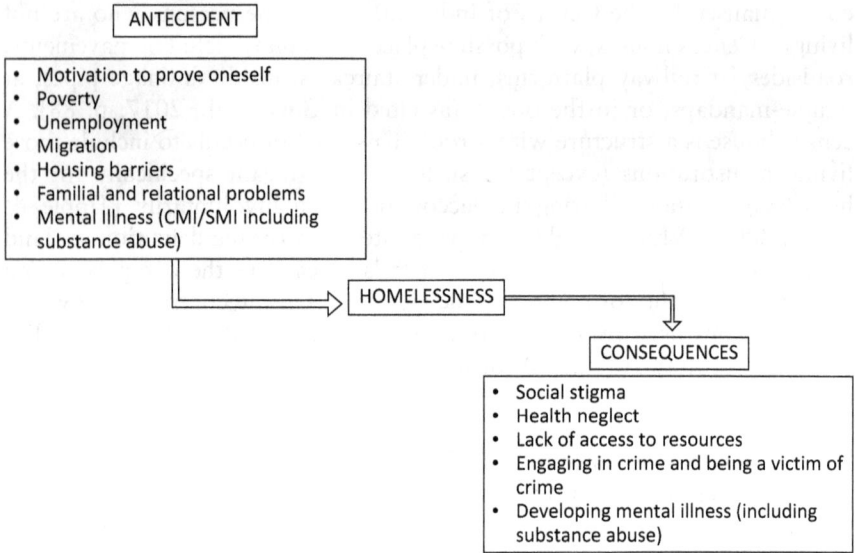

ANTECEDENT

- Motivation to prove oneself
- Poverty
- Unemployment
- Migration
- Housing barriers
- Familial and relational problems
- Mental Illness (CMI/SMI including substance abuse)

HOMELESSNESS

CONSEQUENCES

- Social stigma
- Health neglect
- Lack of access to resources
- Engaging in crime and being a victim of crime
- Developing mental illness (including substance abuse)

Figure 1.1 Antecedents and Consequences of Homelessness and Serious Mental Illness.

Economists globally identify unequal income distribution as one of the grassroots reasons for poverty in India. Toro and Janisse (2004, p. 247) pointed out that there are some differences in the causal pathway between those who are poor in comparison to those who are poor and homeless. For example, poor and homeless people have a more significant share of stressful life experiences, vulnerability to being the victim of domestic and community violence, and disordered background (history of sexual and physical abuse, family history of mental illness, and substance abuse, etc.).

- According to the Centre for Monitoring Indian Economy Pvt Ltd., India's unemployment rate (UPR) during the first quarter of 2022 was 7.43% (7.8% urban UPR, 7.2% rural UPR).[1] *Unemployment* further maintains the poverty level and, as an extension, homelessness. It also affects the migration trajectories within the nation.
- According to a report published by the Ministry of Statistics & Programme Implementation, 10.8% of migrants migrate due to employment-related issues (in search of employment/better employment/to take up employment/to take up better employment/business/proximity to a place of work/transfer/loss of job/closure of unit/lack of employment opportunities).[2] Individuals also migrate due to natural disasters, socio-political reasons, displacement due to developmental projects, etc. However, while migrating due to unemployment, individuals have fewer resources to access adequate shelter and often end up homeless. In a study conducted in Mumbai, Prashad et al. (2016) reported that 38.2% of the urban homeless were from Maharashtra, while the remaining 61.8% were migrants from other states of India.

- With the ever-increasing population growth, rapid urbanisation, and migration, scarcity of accessible and affordable *housing* remains one of the most significant barriers in India

Socio-cultural Factors:

- Within the socio-cultural context of the patriarchal system of India, women are already considered to be more *at risk* than their male counterparts in multiple ways. Domestic violence and intimate partner violence increase these vulnerabilities, including homelessness. Sometimes they are not allowed to stay at home or might be driven to choose homelessness to avoid violence. The assaulters might include their husbands, in-laws, siblings, children, and even parents.
- Even with no apparent violence, interpersonal conflicts within the household might force individuals to leave the conflict zone. Such extreme choices are not uncommon, particularly when the individual cannot get help to deal with conflicts. Lack of social support, financial empowerment, information, accessibility to affordable housing, and poor health conditions might interfere with the availability of help and increase the chance of homelessness.
- The propensity to engage in crime or be a victim of crime increases due to homelessness. Petty crimes like theft, bag-lifting, chain-snatching, and pickpocketing are often committed by young homeless men and children. They often engage in criminal activities through organised rackets (Kulkarni, 2016). While for many, it is a way to survive street life, coming out of the vicious cycle becomes a challenge due to inaccessibility to alternatives.
- Homeless individuals are particularly vulnerable to being assaulted by the police, goons, and community members (Chandran, 2018). Homeless women on the streets are often sexually harassed, which ranges from being molested, and raped by strangers or fellow homeless men, to gang rape (Bhattacharya, 2022). Street children and homeless women with mental illnesses are particularly at risk.

Socio-medical Factors:

- Physical and mental illnesses often result in out-of-pocket spending, directly contributing to increased expenditure, less saving, and increased poverty.
- Living on the streets makes the homeless population more vulnerable to various illnesses due to factors like malnutrition affecting immunity to catching infectious agents, including coronavirus disease-2019 (COVID-19). In addition, lack of public hygiene, inadequate waste disposal, extreme weather conditions, contamination, increased prevalence of infections, and substance abuse contribute significantly to poorer physical and mental well-being.

- National Resource and Training Centre on Homelessness and Mental Illness (2003) estimated that 20–25% of the homeless population suffers from an SMI, even in higher-income countries where resources are more accessible, the treatment gap is smaller, and the population is lesser. Untreated mental health conditions[3] might also increase the chance of homelessness (Gopikumar, Narasimhan et al., 2015, p. 45).

Homelessness and SMI – The Vicious Loop

The literature on homelessness has established poor mental health conditions as both antecedents and consequences of homelessness (Gopikumar, Narasimhan et al., 2015). Homelessness brings along innumerable atrocities. Homelessness becomes devastating when coupled with poor mental health, especially a serious one.

Substance Abuse and Mental Health Service Administration (SAMHSA) in 2012 defined serious mental illnesses as "a group of mental disorders that result in serious functional impairment that substantially interferes with a person's ability to carry out life activities" (as cited in Bonugli et al., 2013, p. 827). It includes specifically schizophrenia, bipolar affective disorder, schizoaffective disorder, and severe depression with psychosis.

Not all homeless people indeed end up having a mental illness; not all individuals who have a mental illness reach the point of homelessness. Nevertheless, the lack of resources makes it more difficult for them to exit it as they are involuntarily expelled by society towards the vicious cycle of homelessness-SMI. However, one might get a chance to develop a new or renewed relational world, for example, through community-based rehabilitation with the help of family, neighbours, or service providers. This community-based rehabilitation may make exiting the cycle of homelessness-SMI possible. Otherwise, the double jeopardy of homelessness and SMI continues in an endless loop. Gopikumar, Narasimhan et al. (2015) pointed out that:

> very few conditions have as debilitating or devastating an effect as the co-occurrence of homelessness and mental illness.... People's mental ill health often robs them of basic survival and self-preservation skills; many are found wandering emaciated, and with wounds that are sometimes infested with maggots.
>
> (pp. 44–45)

Being feared and ignored by a large section of society, the susceptibility of HMI individuals increases manifold. Robbed of their fundamental right and access to resources, living an uncertain life, they are more vulnerable to becoming victims of crime, physical ill-health, and deprivation.

Statistics of HMI Persons – How Severe is the Pan India Epidemic?

Homelessness in India is a complex, multifaceted phenomenon. The statistics of it is also varying to no small extent. While there is the availability of research data on HMI from high-income countries and some Asian countries, there is a general lack of epidemiological data from India. This may be because of the fleeting nature of the population that makes long-term accessibility difficult. The lack of an operational definition also plays a significant obstacle in obtaining epidemiological data. According to the Census of India (2011), India has 1.77 million homeless[4] (Goel et al., 2017), which many researchers consider being under-reporting "due to the lacunae in enumeration" (Sattar, 2014, p. 11). ActionAid, in a survey conducted in 2003, estimated that the homeless population in India is 78 million (Sattar, 2014). This same survey has reported that the number of homeless people is highest in the metro cities of Delhi, Kolkata, Chennai, and Mumbai, respectively. 2011 has marked a decrease in rural homelessness and an increase in urban homelessness. An increased migration rate from villages to cities in search of better employment opportunities and living conditions has played a role in this.

In India, epidemiological surveys report a lifetime prevalence of mental disorders as 9.4–70/1000 population (Malhotra et al., 2013). As per the National Mental Health Survey (NMHS) in 2016, data revealed a vast "mental health gap" of 85.4% and one in five individuals suffering from a mental health disorder. There are 0.75 psychiatrists/1,00,000 Indians compared to 6/1,00,000 in high-income countries (Garg et al., 2019). The NMHS also showed a disproportionate distribution of services, with most resources clustering in urban cities.

Following the trends in higher-income group countries, the National Resource and Training Centre on Homelessness and Mental Illness (2003) estimated that even in such nations where resources are more accessible with lesser treatment gap and lesser population, 20–25% of the homeless population suffers some form of SMI (Gopikumar, Narasimhan et al., 2015, p. 45). For India, assuming this percentage and considering that there are at least 1.77 million homeless as per the Census of India, 2011 (Goel et al., 2017), the estimated number of homeless people suffering SMI becomes on the verge of half a million. Much of this population belongs to urban India.

Mental Health and Illness-Related Studies of HMI Persons in India

Gowda et al. (2017) identified that many homeless individuals with mental illnesses are brought to government-sector hospitals. However, the lack of critical information (personal, family, identification details) poses an unprecedented crisis for medico-legal and humanitarian intervention. To understand the socio-demographic and clinical profile of the HMI persons, they did a retrospective chart review of these patients for the last 13 years (January 2002–31 December 2015) admitted to the Department of Psychiatry at the National Institute of Mental Health and Neurosciences (NIMHANS). Their findings reported that the mean age of the sample was 34.6 years, with more than 50% of female patients. Almost all were registered as medico-legal cases (94.9%), and 80.8% were admitted under court order. HMI patients were brought by police, the public, or NGOs/social workers. Approximately 65.4% of them had schizophrenia, 30.8% had mental retardation, and 29.5% were diagnosed with comorbid substance-use disorder. Health-related complexities like anaemia and malnutrition were found in 43.6% and 32.1% of the patients, respectively.

In a similar study conducted in another government hospital psychiatry unit, Singh et al. (2016) reported that most of the HMI individuals were picked up from the railway station or streets by police, NGOs, or the public. Most of them were below 40 years of age, suffered SMI, and had poor vitals and pregnancy in women. However, with medical intervention, almost all responded to treatment and could be restored to the family once they could remember the address or contact details with the help of NGOs and police.

In a retrospective chart review of HMI persons over six years, Tripathi et al. (2013) reported more than 90.7% having a psychiatric diagnosis with comorbid substance abuse (44.3%), intellectual disabilities (38.6%), and health problems (75.4%). On treatment, 70% could be reintegrated. They identified that "untreated/inadequately treated mental illness was the most common reason for homelessness" (p. 404).

In a recent study on HMI women, Krishnadas et al. (2021) examined the prevalence and factors underlying homelessness. Most women who experienced homelessness had access to treatment, yet they found themselves on the streets. Poor education and disrupted relationships were found to be two leading contributors, primarily rooted in gender-based disadvantage that stopped them from developing a safety net when vulnerable. All these studies (Gowda et al., 2017; Singh et al., 2016; Tripathi et al., 2013) identify the treatment gap in the mental health sector as a leading contributing factor towards mental illness. However, as most of the HMI persons could be found to respond to treatment effectively, these authors suggested providing adequate mental healthcare for the HMI persons through outreach services and collaborative initiatives by governmental and non-governmental organisations (Kaur & Pathak, 2016; Tripathi et al., 2013).

To understand antecedents of the descent into homelessness and to gain insight into approaches that promote personal recovery in institutional care settings amongst HMI persons, Gopikumar, Easwaran et al. (2015) used focus group discussions, interviews, and case histories. They found that along with poverty and unequal income distribution, deprivation, critical life events like the death of the primary caregiver and broken family take away from the person with an SMI the support system. It eventually robs them of a sense of belongingness, rendering them homeless. They further identified "social affiliations, kinship, congruence between the real and ideal self, and the drive to assume a more powerful identity and pursue self-actualisation" as factors facilitating personal recovery (p. 1). Their study further highlights the critical need to explore within an institution the strategies that might help the survivors of homelessness-SMI "pursue well-being," which in turn might promote personal recovery. Moorkath et al. (2018) identified the condition of HMI women in India as more complex as the patriarchal societal norm does not allow women to live or wander on the streets. Once homeless, due to mental illness or otherwise, women are rarely allowed back into the family. Even if they receive medical treatment for their mental illness, they become alienated from their family, friends, or neighbours and end up being in shelter homes for mere survival (p. 477). Through five case studies, they highlight the various familial, individual, economic, societal, and cultural factors that contribute to the phenomenon in women. They have discussed the role of the stigma associated with women with mental illness and women with homelessness as complicating the problem further. They also identified that the beginning of recovery starts with the fundamental essence of hope; however, that is possible only when they are accepted back into society.

HMI Persons' Life within the Hierarchies: Identifying the Gaps of Interest and Beyond

An individual-centric, psychopathology-oriented focus of the existing system limits the understanding of HMI persons through the disability lens. The goal of symptom reduction might prevent stakeholders from looking beyond symptoms. It may hinder the recognition and enhancement of the strengths and resilience of the HMI persons, enabling them to survive extremely hostile environments. A critical review of the literature and the existing mental health policies in India helped identify the gaps of interest.

Impairment-focused understanding of mental health: India signed the United Nations Convention on Rights of Persons with Disabilities (UNCRPD, 2006) in 2007. As identified by the mental health policymakers of the country and activists like Davar (2012), by agreeing to be a part of this convention, India consequently committed to her citizens "its obligation to respect, protect and fulfil the enjoyment of all human rights and freedoms by all people with disabilities, on an equal basis with others" (p. 124). It shifted the policymakers' gaze towards a socio-centric paradigm and the constructs of identity, equality, non-discrimination, and protection of their rights. This initiative is supposed to bridge the gap between the end-users' needs and the erstwhile predominantly clinical recovery-based interventions. A result of this is the Mental Healthcare Act of 2017. The proposed objective of the Mental Healthcare Act (2017) is to

> provide for mental healthcare and services for persons with mental illness and to protect, promote and fulfil the rights of such persons during delivery of mental healthcare and services and for matters connected therewith or incidental thereto.
>
> (p. 1)

On the face of this, the Mental Healthcare Act seems to comply with UNCRPD. It ensures care to individuals in the community setting, which was beyond the scope of the Mental Health Act of 1987. However, the Mental Healthcare Act (2017) defines mental illness as follows:

> a substantial disorder of thinking, mood, perception, orientation, or memory that grossly impairs judgment, behaviour, capacity to recognise reality or ability to meet the ordinary demands of life, mental conditions associated with the abuse of alcohol and drugs but does not include mental retardation which is a condition of arrested or incomplete development of mind of a person, primarily characterised by subnormality of intelligence.
>
> (p. 4)

This is, again, an impairment-only definition. It ignores the personal strengths and resources of the person. It fails to include the person, personal identity, personal recovery, or empowerment as significant research and intervention concerns. Thus, it does not meet the pace of UNCRPD, whose primary concern has been to accommodate the person in the patient. It further fails to capture the disabling aspects of familial, societal, and attitudinal barriers and recognises the equality of people having psycho-social disabilities with people having other physical disabilities but not citizens in general.

Underexplored role of recovery and empowerment: Research in the last three decades has consistently reported a close association of homelessness with mental illness (Bhugra, 2007; Patel & Kleinman, 2003; Susser et al., 1990). The existing literature in India on this population has identified the role of the treatment gap as a contributing and maintenance factor for the homeless population with mental illness. Authors have already suggested the need to explore the role of hope as a factor that might facilitate the recovery process in HMI persons (Gopikumar, Easwaran et al., 2015; Moorkath et al., 2018). Nevertheless, little research has been done to understand the factors that might drive them towards vertical social mobility, that is, a change in their position in an upward direction (upward mobilisation) from the margins to the mainstream.

Inadequate understanding of the context and voice of HMI persons: The possibility of including the context and voice of the HMI person has hardly been the focus of research. Research on any marginalised population demands the representation of their voice in their words. Not our interpretation of their life stories or the activities they resort to survive exorbitantly adverse situations. For example, an HMI woman in ragged clothes and a dishevelled state might not be an expression of her disorganised behaviour owing to psychosis but a strategy to keep herself safe from falling prey to repeated sexual assaults in the streets. Despite that, the diverse situations in which the HMI persons find themselves remain primarily unaccounted for.

The medicalisation of socio-genic distress: Homelessness is primarily a social problem. Even when the homeless person is diagnosed with SMI, we cannot overlook the socio-politico-economical context of it. The medicalisation of it is to see HMI persons in clinical and therapeutic terms. The problem is seen as residing in the individuals; the solution is living in treatment and clinical case management following the medical model. It unnecessarily bounds the range of vulnerabilities we are willing to consider when considering factors that make some marginalised groups more vulnerable than others (Snow et al., 1994). The medical model thus adopts the language of disability. It limits our understanding of these populations.

Thus, we attempt to know little about what might be right with the HMI populations, the strengths that empower them to survive the extremely harsh environment, and the strategies they develop to make ends meet. We do not try to understand if it is the evolutionary instinct of survival of the fittest or their resilience and hope towards a better tomorrow in the face of the adversities that keep them going. The literature has always focused on what is wrong with HMI persons, their mental ill health, substance abuse problems, and their inability to float back into the mainstream. Their undefeatable resilience against the extreme hostility of society remains overlooked in the process.

In keeping with the medicalisation trend of neoliberal capitalist society, service approaches frequently identify people with mental illness as consumers of mental healthcare services. However, service approaches have become pathology-centric instead of identifying and building upon the strengths and resilience of a marginalised population like HMI persons. Such individualised responsibility for illness and recovery, disguised as freedom and agency, has exacerbated the existing marginalisation and alienation as they fight alone for services, amenities, and welfare. In a developing country like India, the struggle to avail the barely enough resources to survive for those living with the double burden of mental illness and homelessness is superimposed upon the pre-existing battle for a healthier physical, social, psychological, and economic existence.

Notes

1 https://unemploymentinindia.cmie.com/.
2 https://pib.gov.in/PressReleaseIframePage.aspx?PRID=1833854.
3 According to World Health Organization "A mental disorder is characterised by a clinically significant disturbance in an individual's cognition, emotional regulation, or behaviour. It is usually associated with distress or impairment in important areas of functioning. There are many different types of mental disorders. Mental disorders may also be referred to as mental health conditions. The latter is a broader term covering mental disorders, psychosocial disabilities, and (other) mental states associated with significant distress, impairment in functioning, or risk of self-harm."
4 It should be noted that these are all pre-COVID-19 data. While no updated census report is available yet, but according to a report published by Reuters in 2020, the

number of homeless in India shot to 4 million plus during the peak of the pandemic lockdown (Siddiqui & Kataria, 2020). However, with the gradual waning of the effect of the pandemic, the official number has fallen back to 1.8 million (https://www.homelessworldcup.org/india).

References

Bandyopadhyay, P. (2014, October 10). হাত বাড়ালেই বন্ধু. Anandabazar.com. Retrieved from https://www.anandabazar.com/amp/supplementary/rabibashoriyo/%E0%A6%B9-%E0%A6%A4-%E0%A6%AC-%E0%A7%9C-%E0%A6%B2-%E0%A6%87-%E0%A6%AC%E0%A6%A8-%E0%A6%A7-1.76009

Bhattacharya, P. (2022). "Nowhere to sleep safe": Impact of sexual violence on homeless women in India. *Journal of Psychosexual Health*, 4(4), 223–226.

Bhugra, D. (Ed.). (2007). *Homelessness and mental health*. Cambridge University Press.

Bonugli, R., Lesser, J., & Escandon, S. (2013). "The Second Thing to Hell is Living Under that Bridge": Narratives of women living with victimization, serious mental illness, and in homelessness. *Issues in Mental Health Nursing*, 34(11), 827–835.

Chandran, R. (2018, August 14). *'Too afraid to sleep': India's homeless women suffer as cities expand*. Reuters. Retrieved December 11, 2022, from https://www.reuters.com/article/us-india-housing-women-idUSKBN1KZ00S

Davar, B. V. (2012). Legal frameworks for and against people with psychosocial disabilities. *Economic & Political Weekly*, 47(52), 123.

Garg, K., Kumar, C. N., & Chandra, P. S. (2019). Number of psychiatrists in India: Baby steps forward, but a long way to go. *Indian Journal of Psychiatry*, 61(1), 104.

Goel, G., Ghosh, P., Ojha, M. K., & Shukla, A. (2017). Urban homeless shelters in India: Miseries untold and promises unmet. *Cities*, 71, 88–96.

Gopikumar, V., Easwaran, K., Ravi, M., Jude, N., & Bunders, J. (2015). Mimicking family like attributes to enable a state of personal recovery for persons with Mental Illness in Institutional Care Settings. *International Journal of Mental Health Systems*, 9(1), 30.

Gopikumar, V., Narasimhan, L., Easwaran, K., Bunders, J., & Parasuraman, S. (2015). Persistent, complex and unresolved issues: Indian discourse on mental ill health and homelessness. *Economic and Political Weekly*, 50(11), 42–51.

Gowda, G. S., Gopika, G., Manjunatha, N., Kumar, C. N., Yadav, R., Srinivas, D., Dawn, B. R., & Math, S. B. (2017). Sociodemographic and clinical profiles of homeless mentally ill admitted in mental health institute of South India: 'Know the Unknown' project. *International Journal* of *Social Psychiatry*, 63(6), 525–531.

Kaur, R., & Pathak, R. K. (2016). Homelessness and mental health in India. *The Lancet Psychiatry*, 3(6), 500–501.

Krishnadas, P., Narasimhan, L., Joseph, T., Bunders, J., & Regeer, B. (2021). Factors associated with homelessness among women: A cross-sectional survey of outpatient mental health service users at The Banyan, India. *Journal of Public Health*, 43(Supplement_2), ii17–ii25.

Kulkarni, S. (2016, February 27). *Pune: "homeless are victims of a vicious cycle of crimes"*. The Indian Express. Retrieved December 11, 2022, from https://indianexpress.com/article/india/india-news-india/pune-homeless-are-victims-of-a-vicious-cycle-of-crimes/

Malhotra, S., Chakrabarti, S., & Shah, R. (2013). Telepsychiatry: Promise, potential, and challenges. *Indian Journal of Psychiatry*, 55(1), 3.

Moorkath, F., Vranda, M. N., & Naveenkumar, C. (2018). Lives without roots: Institutionalized homeless women with Chronic Mental Illness. *Indian Journal of Psychological Medicine*, 40(5), 476.

Patel, V., & Kleinman, A. (2003). Poverty and common mental disorders in developing countries. *Bulletin of the World Health Organization*, 81(8), 609–615.

Pearsall, J. (1999). *The Concise Oxford Dictionary*. Oxford University Press.

Prashad, L., Lhungdim, H., & Dutta, M. (2016). An enquiry into migration and homelessness–a developmental discourse: Evidence from Mumbai City. *International Journal of Innovative Knowledge Concepts*, 2(1), 33–39.

Sattar, S. (2014). Homelessness in India. *Shelter-Hudco Publication*, 15, 9–15.

Siddiqui and Kataria. (2020, March 31). India's homeless stranded by coronavirus lockdown. Retrieved June 21, 2023, from https://www.reuters.com/article/health-coronavirus-india-homeless-idINKBN21J557

Singh, G., Shah, N., & Mehta, R. (2016). The clinical presentation and outcome of the institutionalized wandering mentally ill in India. *Journal of Clinical and Diagnostic Research: JCDR*, 10(10), VC13.

Snow, D. A., Anderson, L., & Koegel, P. (1994). Distorting tendencies in research on the homeless. *The American Behavioral Scientist*, 37(4), 461.

Susser, E., Goldfinger, S. M., & White, A. (1990). Some clinical approaches to the homeless mentally ill. *Community Mental Health Journal*, 26(5), 463–480.

The Mental Healthcare Act. (2017). Retrieved from http://egazette.nic.in/WriteReadData/2017/175248.pdf

Tipple, A. G., & Speak, S. E. (2005). *Homelessness in developing countries*. Newcastle upon Tyne, Global Urban Research Unit, University of Newcastle upon Tyne.

Tipple, G., & Speak, S. (2009). *The hidden millions: Homelessness in developing countries*. Routledge.

Toro, P. A., & Janisse, H. C. (2004). Patterns of homelessness. *Encyclopaedia of homelessness*. Great Barrington, MA: Berkshire Publishing/Sage. [Online]. Available: http://sun.science.wayne.edu/~ptoro/hopats4.pdf. (January 2006).

Tripathi, A., Nischal, A., Dalal, P. K., Agarwal, V., Agarwal, M., Trivedi, J. K., & Arya, A. (2013). Sociodemographic and Clinical Profile of Homeless Mentally Ill Inpatients in a North Indian Medical University. *Asian Journal of Psychiatry*, 6(5), 404–409.

United Nations. (1998). *Principles and recommendation for population and housing censuses*. United Nations.

United Nations. (2006). *Convention on the rights of persons with disabilities*. New York, USA. Retrieved from https://www.un.org/development/desa/disabilities/convention-on-the-rights-of-persons-with-disabilities/convention-on-the-rights-of-persons-with-disabilities-2.html

United Nations Habitat. (2015). *International guidelines on urban and territorial planning*. Nairobi: United Nations Human Settlements Programme.

2 Exploring Voices of Suffering, Recovery, and Empowerment

Theoretical and Methodological Approaches

Radhika Devi, a 50-year-old lady, was diagnosed with a serious mental health condition. She runs a tea stall with the help of an NGO that works with homeless mentally ill (HMI) individuals in Kolkata. She met all the criteria for being a participant in my research. But when I approached her, she refused to give an interview.

> "I do not want to talk to you. I don't like you. You can sit here all day long if you want, but I will not talk to you" said Ms R.G. I was speechless! I did not know how to convince her for the interview. ...This was the first time I got rejected by a potential participant during fieldwork. I felt insulted, my eyes burning. On my way back from the tea-shop to the female shelter-house at Kolkata, I kept pondering on what exactly went wrong! What was so unacceptable in my demeanor that provoked her. After all, I was a qualified clinical psychologist, trained in 'building rapport' and 'breaking ice'. I needed to understand where that 'No' was coming from.
>
> (Pandey et al., 2019, p. 117)

I chose to understand her social and cultural context before jumping to a conclusion. I returned to her file and got some newer insights into her background and worldview, which helped refine my empathic connection with her. I understood that her blatant "No" may be a protest against the structural violence she has been a victim of all her life. I consciously acknowledged the "autonomy" that had been core to her survival. I could realise that I had a choice to initiate exploring the world of a highly vulnerable group. Similarly, she had a choice or resolve not to talk to someone like me who belonged to the "other" world (oppressive state, society, and family) whose hegemony she had been fighting against (Pandey et al., 2019, p. 118).

Radhika's intense "No" was her way of showing her indifference as well as defiance towards the hierarchies that have victimised her. And thus, even her silence had the power to make her voice heard in her way. It was not how I, as a researcher or the society at large, needed her to speak. Even without telling me her story, Radhika became an example for me.

DOI: 10.4324/9781032662053-2

This experience and the gaps I identified in the previous chapter reaffirmed my resolve that a study has long been due in the Indian setting, which would consider the hierarchies that catalysed the process of becoming an HMI person and beyond. Accordingly, the following sections provide a brief understanding of the theoretical and methodological lenses through which I delved into the lived experiences of the HMI persons.

Understanding Psychiatric Rehabilitation Process for HMI Persons within the Framework of Recovery and Empowerment

As elaborated in Chapter 1, the pathology-centric understanding of mental illness and marginalised populations like the homeless has focused on "what-is-not-right" with them. Corrigan et al. (2008), in their book *Principles and Practice of Psychiatric Rehabilitation: An Empirical Approach*, identified a common mistake practised globally in planning rehabilitation for people with psychosocial disabilities. The error is to consider their needs different from and lesser than the norm. At times, their needs are different, but under no circumstances are their needs more secondary. The Mental Healthcare Act (2017) of India also compromised on this by identifying the rights of people with psychosocial disabilities with people with physical disabilities but not the able-bodied citizens.

The Relevance of the Psychiatric Rehabilitation Process in HMI Persons

The recent advances in the practice of psychiatric rehabilitation have witnessed a paradigm shift. Corrigan et al. (2008) posited that the driving goals of psychiatric rehabilitation "fall into the same set of aspirations as those that are a priority for all adults: employment, residence, relationships, and health (both physical and mental)" (p. viii).

In the second edition of their book *Psychiatric Rehabilitation*, Anthony et al. (2002) conceptualised it as the process to "help persons with psychiatric disabilities to increase their ability to function successfully and to be satisfied in the environments of their choice with the least amount of ongoing professional intervention" (p. 101). Rutman (1993) understood it as an opportunity provided to people with psychiatric disabilities "to work, live in the community, and enjoy a social life, at their own pace, through planned experiences in a respectful, supportive, and realistic atmosphere" (as cited in Corrigan et al. 2008, p. 1). This definition highlights that the focus of psychiatric rehabilitation needs to remain grounded in normalising roles and relationships through practical and realistic elements of one's daily life experiences.

It is apparent how resources have been recurrently denied to marginalised populations at familial and systemic levels. It thus becomes more crucial to include and emphasise the concept of recovery and empowerment as there is a paucity of attempts to utilise these concepts and conceptualise a holistic rehabilitation process. Empowerment might entail people with disabilities having power over all aspects of their lives and rehabilitation. This kind of self-determination assures the development of life decisions consistent with a person's overall sense of self. Related to empowerment is the idea of recovery – people with psychosocial disabilities can and do recover (Corrigan et al., 2008, p. ix). A more detailed description of recovery and empowerment follows.

Recovery and Empowerment: The Pillars of Psychiatric Rehabilitation

In their article "The Rediscovery of Recovery: Open to All," the authors Roberts and Wolfson (2004) credited Anthony (1993) to have provided a widely accepted definition of recovery, which involves

> a deeply personal, unique process of changing one's attitudes, values, feelings, goals, skills and roles. It is a way of living a satisfying, hopeful, and contributing life even with limitations caused by the illness. Recovery involves the development of new meaning and purpose in one's life as one grows beyond the catastrophic effects of mental illness.
>
> (p. 39)

Anthony poses that an individual with mental illness can recover even when the symptoms have not subsided, including the disabilities resulting from the symptoms.

Another pivotal pillar of the psychiatric rehabilitation process has been empowerment. The Cornell University Empowerment Group defined empowerment as "an intentional, ongoing process centred in the local community, involving mutual respect, critical reflection, caring and group participation, through which people lacking an equal share of valued resources gain greater access to and control over those resources" (1989, as cited in Zimmerman 2000, p. 43).

A person needs to be adequately empowered to overcome the downward change in their social position (downward mobilisation) that has already taken place and move upwards towards a more socially integrated, purposeful contributing life. A population as alienated as the HMI individuals is marked by an absence of home, family, kin, or kith to care for them. Therefore, they rely on the community and the service providers to gain access and control with the necessary socio-economical and other resources.

One will not be searching for the valued resources for being empowered if one does not have hope, purpose, and meaning in life. Living an empowered life is not possible when one lacks valued resources. Recovery and empowerment, therefore, are complementary to each other for a marginalised population like the HMI persons. Rediscovering valued personal resources helps one gain access and control over other valuable resources. Therefore, it becomes an immensely critical concern when one targets psychiatric rehabilitation, especially for suchmarginalised populations like the HMI persons, who cannot exit the vicious cycle of homelessness–SMI because of this lack of resources.

Challenges to Recovery and Empowerment in HMI Persons

The accessibility to resources for marginalised populations like HMI persons is scarce. It has been denied at every fundamental level (familial or systemic). And that is where the subjective experience of suffering crosses its threshold and becomes "social suffering." In their seminal work on "Social Suffering," Kleinman et al. (1997) posited, "Social suffering result from what political, economic, and institutional power does to people and, reciprocally, from how these forms of power themselves influence responses to social problems" (p. ix). That various socio-economic and political forces and institutional powers as stakeholders have induced suffering in populations like these cannot be argued more. More ironically, familial and relational processes play a paradoxical bidirectional role. The familial and relational processes induce suffering and share the pain and suffering associated with the illness and marginalisation. Kleinman (2010) has pointed out that the boundary between health problems and social atrocities gets blurred at some point for marginalised populations. Social suffering as a theory helps us to take a perspective "by framing conditions that are both, and that require both health and social policies" (p. 1519).

For centuries, SMIs like schizophrenia have been feared as the "kiss of death" diagnosis (Summerville, n.d., Your Recovery Journey, para. 2). They have been thought to ruin every plan for the future the person made and surrender to the symptoms and assume the role of a helpless patient for the rest of the life. The paradigmatic shift in understanding mental illness and moving beyond the medical model has given space to more meaningful constructs that would help the individual garner hope and transcend the disabilities and identity of a patient. It might further aid them in pursuing the future they always wanted to have. Thus, recovery and empowerment become immensely crucial as psychiatric rehabilitation continues to mature holistically.

The Methodological Lens of Exploring Voices of Suffering, Recovery, and Empowerment

Positioning from the gaps of interest established in the previous chapter, in the following chapters, I would delve into lived experiences of individuals who have survived both homelessness and SMI, adopting the theoretical framework of recovery and empowerment within the purview of psychiatric rehabilitation. In doing so, I explored the following four areas through their life stories: their experiences of social suffering associated with the downward mobilisation, the challenges experienced in their journey towards recovery and empowerment, their experiences of the process of recovery and empowerment, and the experience of service providers in facilitating the process of recovery and empowerment. To this end, using the social constructionism paradigm[1] and critical ethnography[2] methodology, I conducted semi-structured interviews with rehabilitated HMI persons[3] and their service providers[4] at two NGO shelter houses in Kolkata and Chennai.

According to the Census of India (2001), Kolkata had the country's highest homeless population (Sattar, 2014). However, due to practical and ethical constraints, it was impossible to reach out to the HMI people residing on the streets. I was to take the help of gatekeepers who would help me access the field. Gatekeepers are the entry-point contact with control over critical sources and avenues of opportunity within the field. I entered the field with the help of the NGO Iswar Sankalpa in Kolkata.

Chennai was the other city where I conducted the second phase of the fieldwork; the setting, in this case, was chosen following the formulation of the research problem because it could accommodate the requirements of the research goal. According to a survey conducted by ActionAid International, Chennai has the third-highest population of homeless individuals following Delhi and Kolkata. That said, the mere support of statistics was insufficient to narrow down the field. As mentioned earlier, having the right gatekeeper plays a significant role. Of all the NGOs working in India with this population (the number is meagre, Kolkata, Chennai, Mumbai, Guwahati, and Goa, one in each of these cities), I got permission from three. However, one of them withdrew their consent later, leaving it to Kolkata and Chennai. The NGO, The Banyan, was my gatekeeper in Chennai during my fieldwork. The fieldwork was conducted in four intermediate phases (three to four months, twice in both NGOs) between August 2016 and March 2018.

Besides interviews, data were collected through participant observations and taking field notes. The interviews were conducted in their natural settings, either at the shelter homes, shared houses, or in the community. These interactions were audio-recorded, transcribed verbatim, and then analysed using the constructionist grounded theory (CGT) methodology.[5]

I will present schematically here for a technical understanding of the critical insights gained through these analyses revolving around the four areas I intended to explore. For a detailed understanding of the same, refer to their operational definitions in Appendix III. Now, I assure the readers that while it may read quite dry and filled with jargon, these definitions come in handy when you explore the life stories of the HMI individuals in the following three chapters.

Though the categories mentioned in Figures 2.1–2.3 appear to be presented chronologically, they were not always linear or sequential within one interview and often overlapped. Moreover, not all the participants experienced all the categories. In the following three chapters, I present 15 life stories of HMI individuals[6].

Before Homelessness-SMI   During/Following Homelessness-SMI

**Exclusion and Victimisation due
to Patriarchal Power Process**

- being victim of domestic violence
- denial of experience and role of
  motherhood
- being victim to patriarchal
  practices
- being victim to exploitations
  based on gender norms
- being victim of poverty and
  unemployment

SMI---Homelessness--HMI

Pathway to HMI

Homelessness—SMI--HMI

Lived-experience of Homelessness

- suffering associated with experiencing
  homelessness
- surviving homelessness
- meaning of home and homelessness

Lived-experience of SMI

- meaning of symptoms and suffering
  associated with SMI
- double jeopardy of being unaware of and
  apathetic nature of service-provision
- consequences of suffering SMI
- ✓ experience of losses due to SMI
- ✓ being a victim of stigma

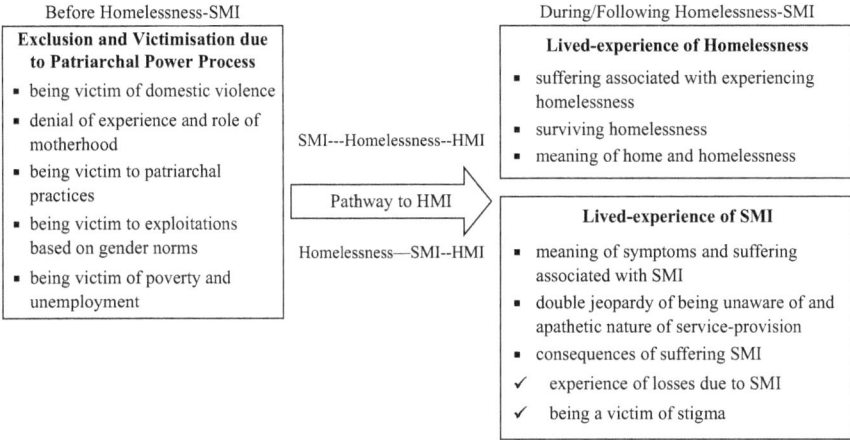

Figure 2.1 Experience of Social Suffering Associated with the Downward Mobilisation.

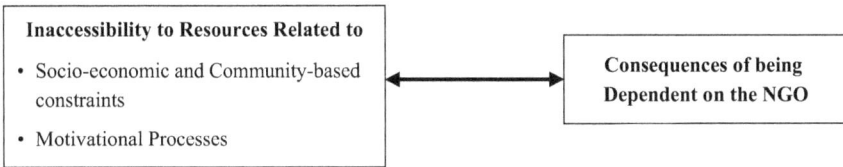

Inaccessibility to Resources Related to

- Socio-economic and Community-based
  constraints
- Motivational Processes

**Consequences of being
Dependent on the NGO**

Figure 2.2 Challenges to the Process of Recovery and Empowerment.

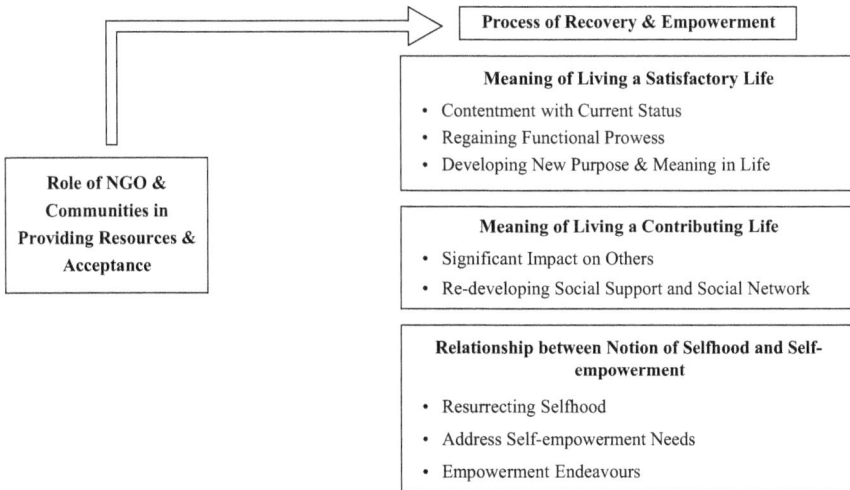

Process of Recovery & Empowerment

Meaning of Living a Satisfactory Life

- Contentment with Current Status
- Regaining Functional Prowess
- Developing New Purpose & Meaning in Life

**Role of NGO &
Communities in
Providing Resources &
Acceptance**

Meaning of Living a Contributing Life

- Significant Impact on Others
- Re-developing Social Support and Social Network

**Relationship between Notion of Selfhood and Self-
empowerment**

- Resurrecting Selfhood
- Address Self-empowerment Needs
- Empowerment Endeavours

Figure 2.3 Process of Recovery and Empowerment.

In Chapter 3, I reauthor the narratives of those individuals who could not overcome the immense social suffering induced by patriarchal power processes or motivational and relational dynamics of old age. Chapter 4 comprises life stories of survivors of homelessness–SMI who initially their life as an HMI person could overcome intense social suffering, but due to the absence of hope, they lost the zeal with which they had started upon the journey and instead chose to be content with their present status in life. Nevertheless, they shared experiences indicate traces of recovery and empowerment. Chapter 5 consists of the reconstructed narratives of those HMI persons who could garner hope as a way of life through their relationships with significant others or self-reflections on their experiential journeys contributing towards experiences of recovery and empowerment despite the hurdles of a multitude of social suffering.

Chapter 6 discusses the experience of service providers in the context of the factors of motivation and challenges. Then, in Chapter 7, I discuss how the previous four chapters could address the context-based rehabilitation issues besides the theoretical gaps in the study of the mental health experiences of HMI individuals. Finally, I discuss some critical theoretical, methodological, applied, and policy-related implications of exploring the lived experiences of HMI persons.

Notes

1 According to Lincoln et al. (2018), social constructionism is the new paradigm of inquiry that has emerged because of the increasing dissatisfaction with the over-emphasis on quantification. As a paradigm, it provides space for the voice of the "researched" within their socio-historical and cultural context. The researcher mirrors the voice of a passionate participant (Lincoln, 1991), "actively engaged in facilitating the 'multi-voice' reconstruction" (Guba & Lincoln, 1994). Locating my theoretical standpoint as that of social constructionism ensured that the voice of my research participants would be heard in the way they wanted themselves to be heard, not the way I wanted them to speak (Sampson, 1993). The social constructionist paradigm could rightfully provide the conceptual window to explore recovery and empowerment within the purview of psychiatric rehabilitation to understand the lived experiences of individuals who have survived both homelessness and serious mental illness.

2 Ethnography allows the researcher understand people's worldviews from their vantage point (Hammersley & Atkinson, 2007). Advocating for the marginalised population against systemic and societal oppression, the ethnographer brings a critical and analytical approach to the research. Critical Ethnography, thus, appeared to be a suitable choice as a qualitative methodology in addressing the questions I wanted to explore centred on reconstructing the lived experience of HMI persons.

3 Life story interviews were conducted with individuals who met the following criteria: individuals (≥18 years) who at some point in their lives have been homeless; those currently living at a shelter house/rehabilitated into the community under the supervision of professionals (psychiatrist/psychologist) or non-professional caregivers/proxy-caregivers; those with a diagnosis of schizophrenia/bipolar affective disorder/schizoaffective disorder/depression with psychotic symptoms

according to ICD-10-DCR criteria (WHO, 1993); but no active psychotic symptoms (in remission) and declared fit for the study by the treating psychiatrist/clinical psychologist/psychiatric social worker and they provided informed consent to be interviewed. However, I did not mention the specific diagnosis the vignettes received since the "label" had no direct impact on re-storying their lived experiences. Nevertheless, a proper diagnosis was one of the most critical steps towards recovery (clinical and personal) for all of them. In this context, I would like to mention that biomedical understanding and psychosocial underpinnings are more complementary than antagonistic; however, their intersections are the "tricky paths". How we tread these paths depends on the approach towards a "disorder" and those affected by it. I firmly acknowledge the critical need for adequate diagnosis and pharmacological therapy for an individual suffering the distress associated with the symptoms of SMI. It is immensely critical for service providers, thus to identify and adapt to the needed service approach for the service user instead of embarking on a journey of proving theoretical propositions.

4 Service providers involved with treatment/rehabilitation/caregiving of HMI individuals as trained mental health professionals/non-technical caregivers/proxy-caregivers with more than five years of working experience. The service providers are the basic social support that HMI individuals have in their existing ecosystem who have the potential to both facilitate as well as obstruct the process of recovery and empowerment. It thus becomes relevant to understand the perspectives, experiences, and challenges that the service providers undergo in working with this population.

5 As an analytical method, the strategies of CGT help to arrange, compile, and gain insights into the collected data in a more holistic way, increasing the "analytic incisiveness" (Charmaz & Mitchell, 2001). Following the transcribing, the data, when ready to be analysed, is coded first. Charmaz (2006, p. 43) conceptualised coding as "categorising segments of data with a short name that simultaneously summarises and accounts for each piece of data. Your codes show how you select, separate, and sort data to begin an analytic accounting of them." A typical CGT analysis would include two types of coding, initial, focused and sometimes axial coding. Charmaz (2006, p. 46) defined initial coding as "naming each word, line, or segment of the data." Focused coding decides "which initial codes make the most analytic sense to categorise your data incisively and completely" (Charmaz, 2006, p. 58).

6 All and any names of HMI individuals used throughout the book are pseudonyms.

References

Anthony, W. A., Cohen, M. R., Farkas, M. D., & Gagne, C. (2002). *Psychiatric Rehabilitation: Center for Psychiatric Rehabilitation*. Boston, MA: Sargent College of Health and Rehabilitation Sciences Boston University.

Charmaz, K. (2006). *Constructing grounded theory: A practical guide through qualitative research*. Sage.

Charmaz, K., & Mitchell, R. G. (2001). Grounded theory in ethnography. In P. Atkinson, A. Coffey, S. Delamont, J. Lofland, & L. H. Lofland (Eds.), *Handbook of ethnography* (pp. 160–174). Sage.

Corrigan, P. W., Mueser, K. T., Bond, G. R., Drake, R. E., & Solomon, P. (2008). *Principles and practice of psychiatric rehabilitation: An empirical approach*. Guilford Press.

Guba, E., & Lincoln, Y. (1994). Competing paradigms in qualitative research. In N. K. Denzin & Y. S. Lincoln (Eds.), *Handbook of qualitative research* (pp. 105–117). Sage.

Hammersley, M., & Atkinson, P. (2007). *Ethnography: Principles in practice.* Routledge.

Kleinman, A. (2010). Four social theories for global health. *The Lancet, 375*(9725), 1518–1519.

Kleinman, A., Das, V., Lock, M., & Lock, M. M. (Eds.). (1997). *Social suffering.* University of California Press.

Lincoln, Y. S. (1991). The detached observer and the passionate participant: Discourses in inquiry and science. In *Annual meeting of the American Educational Research Association*, Chicago.

Lincoln, Y. S., Lynham, S. A., & Guba, E. G. (2018). Paradigmatic controversies, contradictions, and emerging confluences, revisited. In N. K. Denzin, & Y. S. Lincoln (Eds.), *The Sage Handbook of qualitative research* (5th ed., pp. 108–150). Sage.

Pandey, R., Khanna, A., Sharma, D., Gupta, A., Bhattacharya, P., Kukreja, S., & Priya, K. R. (2019). Getting close to the context and experience of illness: Critically reflexive fieldwork in Qualitative Health Research. *Journal of Health Studies, 1*(1), 96–127.

Roberts, G., & Wolfson, P. (2004). The rediscovery of recovery: Open to all. *Advances in Psychiatric Treatment, 10*(1), 37–48.

Sampson, E. E. (1993). Identity politics: Challenges to psychology's understanding. *American Psychologist, 48*(12), 1219.

Sattar, S. (2014). Homelessness in India. *Shelter-Hudco Publication, 15*, 9–15.

Summerville, C. (n.d.). Your Recovery Journey. Retrieved February 7, 2020, from https://www.schizophrenia.ca/your_recovery_journey.php

The Mental Healthcare Act. (2017). Retrieved from http://egazette.nic.in/WriteReadData/2017/175248.pdf

World Health Organization. (1993). *The ICD-10 classification of mental and behavioural disorders: diagnostic criteria for research* (Vol. 2). World Health Organization.

Zimmerman, M. A. (2000). Empowerment theory. In J. Rappaport & E. Seidman (Eds.), *Handbook of community psychology* (pp. 43–63). Springer Science & Business Media.

3   The Suffering of the Forgotten Voices

The gradual transcendence in mental health research beyond the medical model has given scope and space for more meaningful concepts like recovery and empowerment for the intervention. As already elaborated in Chapter 1, individuals with homelessness and SMI (HMI) remain one of the worst affected sections of the human population globally. Through their life stories, I attempt to explore how a marginalised population like HMI persons survives such an extreme paucity of resources; and how they face those challenges to recovery and empowerment.

However, not all tales of HMI persons are about the experiences of recovery or empowerment. Not all of them emerge victoriously, breaking the vicious cycle. On the contrary, some remain stuck in the maze of suffering, losing their way for various reasons. But then, why do I need to tell these stories if they are not the stories of recovery or empowerment? It is because these stories would celebrate the abilities of these people to tolerate all forms of ostracisation yet never flee from life and endure the sufferings with immense fortitude!

The first two stories in this chapter are of "Ruhi," from Bangladesh, and "Kavita," from Gujarat. Both had been victims of the patriarchal power processes all their life, betrayed, and denounced by familial relations and failed by society. Stuck in two parts of India for various systemic reasons (Ruhi in Kolkata and Kavita in Chennai), both the stories reverberate the intense hopelessness gathered over these experiences and the challenges they face in looking beyond the bleak grey that life appeared to them.

Next, I present the stories of "Lavanya," "Muraad," and "Nalini." All three had lived their youth fighting against the suffering that life kept throwing their way. They were in their late sixties or early seventies when I interviewed them. They felt tired of struggling with the same intensity they had been fighting or striving for a dignified life in their younger days. Looking back, they felt more hopeless when they saw those empty credit columns of the past. Burdened with the "not so unusual ageing problems," with no one to look forward to, they didn't feel like fighting any longer and accepted the inevitable.

DOI: 10.4324/9781032662053-3

Ruhi

Born in Bangladesh, Ruhi was 20 years old when I met her for the first time. It was in August 2016 at Kolkata's female shelter house, "Sarbari." I interacted with her over a cup of *chai* or two, trying to become the "insider." She was training to learn the use of a sewing machine at that time. Some appreciation for her newly found skill was all that I needed to build a rapport, and she was ready to share her life story with me.

Over the next few weeks, we would talk incessantly, in and out of our scheduled interview sessions. Ruhi entrusted me with her deepest secrets and most dreaded fears; she looked forward to my daily visit to the NGO. Whenever she found me, she would talk to me about anything and everything. The trust grew substantially with my multiple visits over the next few years.

Aspects of Social Suffering Associated with the Process of "Becoming"
HMI Person Shaped by Familial and Socio-political Context

Ruhi had been having the dehumanised experience of oppression and humiliation by patriarchal power processes for as long as she could remember. It all started with her mother being victimised by the same power processes.

> My mother was a lovely woman who took care of all household chores. My father gave *talaq* (divorce) to my mother. My mother's elder brother lived in a foreign country. My father asked him to find a job for him there because he had married my mother. My uncle could not. And for that, my father used to beat her severely. He married my mother for money and that job. He drove her crazy. After she became "*pagol*" (mad),[1] my grandfather took her back to his place.

And as an infant, Ruhi became the "collateral damage" to this marital dispute.

> I lived with my mother until I was breastfeeding. Then my uncles took my mother and left me with my father. They were not ready to take care of me. They were to marry and have children of their own. Won't I be a burden to them then!

However, her own experiences of growing up were not much different from her mother's. Her feelings of alienation, dejection, and being a burden to her primary caregivers intensified when her father remarried.

> He said he wanted me to grow up and have an education. But I used to think, why did you marry if you had wished for that? You could have taken care of me, sent me to school, look after my well-being. But he did not do that.

She also was harshly disciplined even for the slightest mistakes

> My father was very aggressive with me. He would beat me with or without reason. One day, I was very young, and we sat to have dinner. I had forgotten to wash my hand before eating. For that, my father threw a brass glass on my forehead. I bled like anything. He was very short-tempered.

Thus, when Ruhi got sexually violated for the first time in her teenage within the safety of her own home by a male relative, she knew better not to tell anyone. She knew that her family would blame her because of being a girl. However, when it happened again, she disclosed it to her grandparents, expecting a supportive reaction. But the norm is the norm. "I ran back to my grandmother. I was terrified. I told my grandparents what had happened. But when my grandfather told my uncle, he started beating me. No one stopped him," she recollected.

Feeling betrayed and dehumanised on being exploited and denied justice even by the caregivers, Ruhi chose to take charge of her own life. She left "home" forever that night, leading to her homelessness. Ruhi left home, hoping to live life according to her terms. But living on the streets was far from what she could hardly imagine, primarily because she was the "vulnerable and weaker sex." On the very first night, she got a hint of that.

> I knew nothing there. I asked people about the way to the railway station. I reached there, got on a random train, and got down at one station. There I found some people selling spinach on the side of the streets. I went and sat there. They took pity on me and gave me a place to sleep. It was late at night. I realised that they were brokers for prostitution. I somehow managed to come out of that place and reached Dhaka.

That was just the beginning of the life ahead, shaped by numerous sexual abuse, pregnancy resulting from that, and her psychological breakdown leading to SMI. Soon, she became the victim of human trafficking and found herself working as a prostitute on the other side of the border in New Delhi. Then, mere luck paved her way to Kolkata, where she was rescued from the streets by Iswar Sankalpa in 2011 in a disorganised and dishevelled state.

Ruhi had tried to find her long-lost mother in other women's care and shelter all her life. First, her stepmother, then her grandmother, and later a community member who gave her refuge during her pregnancy. The meaning of motherhood symbolised unconditional love, care, and security for her. Thus, even when she had her first chance to have her "own family" following the birth of her daughter, her motherly instincts (she was hardly 16) guided her to give up her daughter to a Christian orphanage. She knew she had no resources to provide her daughter with the care and safety the child deserved. And thus,

I was on the streets when some sisters from a Christian hospital took us with them. I told them I would not be able to care for my daughter, and they took my daughter. Again, those voices asked me to run away from that place.

However, these experiences have not altered her meaning of home, which was still embedded in "being with the family." Without that, she found herself homeless. Home for her meant "Where I can live with my mother, my grand-parents, and my daughter." Nevertheless, she knew she could never have a home for herself in the way she would like, "I need no family. I have had enough of it. I do not want to dream about all those things. I want to survive on my own, respectfully—nothing more than that" [her voice choked].

Ruhi acknowledged the immense help she received from Iswar Sankalpa. The social workers from Iswar Sankalpa brought her from the streets to their shelter house. She recollected,

(At Kolkata) I lived under a bridge where many other people were also staying. You feel safer when you are among many people than staying alone. But some of them tried to harass me over there. They tried to do "bad things" (*kharap kaj*) with me. (Social workers) brought me from here from the streets. After I came here, initially, I would not work and would keep to myself. I used to become very angry at times. I heard voices speaking to me—Manorama di (non-professional caregiver) would give me the medicines. I was feeling better gradually.

She could experience and identify the changes she was undergoing when the symptoms subsided. It was the first step towards her recovery.

Challenges to the Process of Recovery and Empowerment

While "feeling better" emotionally, she took seriously ill physically. She was diagnosed with tuberculosis and underwent surgery. However, she "com-plained" to me that though the doctor asked her not to do much work fol-lowing her operation, she was assigned chores like all other residents. She was also made to take care of her regular activities, like washing her clothes and dishes. (When I clarified this with the caregivers, they said it was done with the doctor's permission.) However, the emotionally deprived girl identi-fied this as "not being cared for."

No one washed my clothes for me. I had to do that myself, even the dishes. Will you be able to do this work when you are so sick? If some-one hears me telling you all this, they will scold me. I do not tell anyone about my feelings for that reason. I keep them all to myself! [By this time, she was almost sobbing, tears rolling uncontrollably. She tried in vain to wipe them off!].

I had to assure her that these discussions would remain confidential and that I would be discreet even if I needed to discuss any part of it with her counsellors, and thus, she continued.

> I like to work, but I feel weak all the time. What can I do? I work as long as I afford. But if I lie down for a while when I am tired, they (NGO caregivers) start shouting at me like anything, "She just wants to sit and eat." But that is not true. So I end up arguing and misbehaving with them. I do not want to misbehave, but what can I do when they accuse me without reason?

In some prior incidents, I observed Ruhi arguing with the caregivers, particularly the vocational trainers. There was a "lack of understanding" on the part of the service providers, at least in how they communicated. However, I chose to address this issue and give Ruhi some other choices than ending up "arguing and misbehaving" as she did not enjoy being aggressive. We did a pros-cons analysis of her behaviour together. She identified them, and I wrote them down for her. After doing a role-play of one particular incident, we could see how the conversation could have had a productive ending with some subtle changes in her assertion. I later discussed it with her counsellor with her consent, and we decided to introduce assertiveness training in her sessions. On a different occasion, I was told that Ruhi found it helpful in her daily interaction.

However, she chose to remain distant from her co-residents. She was afraid of being judged. She felt unheard due to a lack of space for her voice within the hierarchical system of the NGO. The first time she felt heard in years was during this conversation, and she ensured that I listened to her right.

> I do not t share anything with anyone. I would do whatever they (caregivers) ask me to do as long as my health permits. Nothing beyond that. What would I get telling them? If I tell them anything, they would say go to the doctor. And what would he do? He would give some more medicines. Are medicines the solution to everything? Does not one need people to talk, share their feelings, go out, and spend time in the open? Most days, we are locked inside these four walls. I have been struggling ever since I remember. My father tortured me so severely when I was a child. Even now, I try to work as much as I can. I have been asked not to do this work after the operation. But still, I need to do them. Here, they give us good food, medicines, and clothes. That's fine. But whatever we earn by working so hard (they receive an allowance for doing the chores at the shelter house) goes to the bank. They say it is for our good. But sometimes, even we would want money in cash to buy things we like. You people are rich; you have enough money in your life. So, it does not matter to you. But it matters to us. We would be asked so many questions, even if we asked for ten rupees from our account. I feel angry.

Her unheard voice vented her frustration, her helplessness, and hopeless-ness. Ruhi reflected the feeling of being dehumanised first by the family, then by society, and now by the hierarchical system of the NGO. Ruhi real-ised that access to the resources came with the cost of giving up her inde-pendence and complying with the rules of the shelter house. Moreover, she knew the NGO was making almost all her decisions on her behalf, which frustrated her.

It had been seven years since she left home. It was the only choice she had made all her life. In hindsight, she could not decide whether it was right, but her family had not left her with many options. The rest were "imposed" upon her without consent by society and the system. Finally, after being stuck in a foreign land due to bureaucratic red tape for seven years, last year, Iswar Sankalpa could successfully repatriate Ruhi to Bangladesh (Bandyopadhyay, 2018). She was sent to stay with an NGO. Again, however, it was not much of her "choice," but what the socio-political system decided to be the "right thing" for her. And once again, she was not heard. Once, during one of her hour-long interactions, I asked Ruhi, "Where do you get the strength to fight all the odds that you have come across?" She smirked, "I do not know. God has never helped me. I just tolerated it. I do not know for what, but I tolerated it."

Ruhi's was one such story where she had no option but to tolerate the endless suffering life had given her. Though she did not realise it, her strength was her "ability to tolerate" and never give up. She had not been living a satisfying, hopeful, or meaningful life. She was neither directly contributing to others' experiences nor empowered. Nevertheless, she kept her head above water, and thus it became essential for me to tell her story here.

Kavita

A resident of Baroda, Gujarat, Kavita, ended up being in Chennai due to HMI. The culture, food, language, everything was as alien to her as they were to me, a Bengali. And thus, we ended up creating a bond that helped me survive all those months and provided her with a space to vent her agony accumulated through her life experiences.

Aspects of Social Suffering Associated with the Process of "Becoming" HMI Person Shaped by Familial and Socio-political Context

Kavita grew up in a conservative socio-economically middle-class family with her parents, four siblings, uncles, and aunts. Very early in life, she real-ised that all the resources available to her brothers would not be provided to her or her sister based on gender norms.

> I was quite proficient in my studies. I used to score almost 80%. But my parents did not let me study after the tenth. Girls study very little in our

society. My sister also stopped going to school after the tenth. We wanted to, but we were not allowed to. My brothers, however, did not like it. So they studied until the tenth and joined my father's business. He had a travel company.

Withholding the feeling of being betrayed, she engaged in the household chores after leaving school, primarily because her ailing mother could not do much of them. Finally, when Kavita reached her "marriageable age," her parents tried to get her married off. However, once again, Kavita became a victim of the existing cultural norms of our patriarchal society that had its parameters for feminine beauty. And having a "dark complexion," Kavita did not match their parameter and was denied her right and choice to get married.

> I never got married. My parents tried to get me married initially, but time passed. Boys used to come with their families to see me; four/five families came. But they all used to reject me because I was dark-complexioned. My parents gave up on me after some time. Instead, they got my sister married. I stayed at home, continuing to do the household work.

Though humiliated by these dehumanising experiences, Kavita could not express them but suppressed all her feelings and suffered alone.

> I used to think that I, too, should have gotten married. Had I been married, I need not have had to witness a day like this. Instead, my sister got married, all my friends got married, and only I was left unmarried. I feel bad for myself. I used to cry alone.

Her loneliness intensified when her mother passed away, and her emotional distress intensified with time.

> After my mother passed away, I used to feel very lonely. I would always stay in my room and cry and talk to myself. I was afraid that people were trying to harm me. I was scared of coming out of the room. My aunt took care of me, and my father took me to a doctor. I had medicine for a year.

She started "feeling better" with regular medication, but Kavita stopped her medication without consultation with the doctor. The lack of awareness of the family members also played a role. Thus, she experienced similar distress when her father died two years later. Again, her siblings sought treatment for her, but this time also, she stopped the medication as soon as she started feeling better.

To keep Kavita engaged after her father's death, her friends found her a job at a local nursery school. Kavita immensely enjoyed her post, not only for the money she earned but for the company of the toddlers. Moreover, it helped her quench her thirst for becoming a mother. But unfortunately, this dream had remained unfulfilled due to further victimisation by patriarchal power practices.

> I had to look after the children, and I liked it. I loved being with children. It was a nursery school, so the children were all 3-4 years old. I wanted to stay among them. I like the way they talked, that babble. I had to take them to the washroom, look after them, and make tea for the teachers. I worked there for one year [her eyes twinkle, and her face lights up as she talks about the children].

Following her father's death, Kavita's uncle now considered himself the head of the family. He disapproved of her working independently and getting financial empowerment.

> My uncle was very much against it. He did not want me to work and would stop me from going to school. Then also I used to give him all the money I earned. I saw him as my father. But he forced me to leave the job.

He forced her to quit the job and made her do as many household chores as possible. In addition, she was being subjected to severe physical and emotional abuse regularly by him.

> My uncle (father's brother) used to beat me. Others used to stop him, but he would not listen. He wanted me to stay at home and work as a maid. I did most of the work, but he would still beat me. Previously he was afraid of my father as he was older than my uncle. But after my father's death, he listened to no one.

It gradually crossed her tolerance threshold, and Kavita repeatedly tried to kill herself, committing suicide.

> I even tried killing myself twice, once by hanging myself and once by drinking mosquito repellent. Both times my aunt stopped me and saved my life. I did not want to live without my parents [tears rolled down].

Since she survived her suicidal attempts, Kavita thought she had no other way but to suffer this inhumane treatment towards her all her life. Eventually, she could not even find the motivation to protest against him.

For her uncle, Kavita thus became the usual way of disposing of his anger and frustration against anybody. On one such event, after a family dispute, he started beating her as usual without any reason. Other family members tried and failed to stop him. That night, it crossed the threshold of her tolerance. After years of being tortured, Kavita left home that night.

I left home that night and boarded a train. I had some money saved. I did not know where I was going or where the train would go! The train stopped here in Chennai. I started living on the streets. I used to beg at a temple, and they gave me prasad. I slept in that compound. It felt safer there.

Kavita did not remember much of her life spent on the streets of Chennai, except that after a few months, she was rescued from there by the NGO in a dishevelled state.

Challenges to the Process of Recovery and Empowerment

Kavita acknowledged the help received from the NGO. Still, she found it challenging to adjust to the different cultures that the NGO had because of being in Tamil Nadu.

I do not like it here. The madams and sirs are good, but I do not want to stay here. I cannot speak Tamil, so I cannot talk with the other girls. I want to go back home. Everything is very different here, language, food. I cannot speak to anyone throughout the day, month after month.

Irrespective of all the dehumanising experiences she accumulated at home, she still could not perceive the shelter house as home. To her, home meant being with her family, and only that could bring her joy. Kavita was ready to compromise to every possible extent to be with her family, even with her uncle, who had tormented her to homelessness. She was prepared to be "imprisoned" back at "home" than in this foreign place. "I think I was better off at home. Once I return, I would do all the household chores. I would just stay home but not here."

Despite all the traumatising experiences, she considered "home" safer than the outside world. Her biggest fear among everything was dying alone, away from her relatives. And that was why she wanted to return to them (at the least to Gujarat) by any means.

The world outside is worse than my uncle's. I hear all the stories of how girls have been raped and killed. At least I was safe at home. If I die here, it will not make any difference to anyone. But if I die at home, at least my sisters-in-law and my aunt would cry over my death. I am terrified of dying here alone.

She had suffered the patriarchal power processes all her life. Her gendered identity, cumulated with SMI and homelessness, had denied her almost everything one could expect from life. Kavita felt that life had been unfair to her. Had there been no illness or homelessness, she could have had experiences as "usual" as any of us.

My life could have been like yours. You have your parents, siblings, and a job. You have studied so much. I, too, wanted to explore and learn. I wish I could study and become a doctor like you, have a life like yours [sighs!].

With nothing and no one to look forward to in her immediate future, Kavita found it difficult to remain hopeful of the days to come. Nevertheless, she chose to face life and live one day at a time.

Lavanya

Lavanya had been a resident of The Banyan for the last 20 years since they started serving the HMI population. An honour graduate in English and Library Science with multiple work experiences to her accolade, she has been managing the file room for The Banyan ever since. However, while life at The Banyan had given her some solace compared to what she had suffered before, it could not provide her with the meaning and hope she had lost to all those atrocities.

Aspects of Social Suffering Associated with the Process of "Becoming" HMI Person Shaped by Familial and Socio-political Context

Lavanya grew up with her sisters amidst very punitive parenting during her childhood. Academically proficient, after completing graduation in English and Library Science, Lavanya bagged a job at the Madras Gymkhana Club. She soon left her parents' home and found accommodation at a ladies' hostel. Self-sufficiency and self-dependency had been her stronghold from the beginning.

> I have done two degrees, one in English and another in Library Science. However, my father and mother tortured me like anything, so I left them. I went to live at a ladies' hostel and found a job at Gymkhana Club. I worked there for six years.

She fell in love and decided to get married during this time. But unfortunately, her parents did not support her choice, and she went against their will to marry this person. Little did she know what was awaiting ahead. Soon she realised that she had been played upon for her money and that her alcoholic husband was an adulterer.

> My husband was a drunkard. He married me only because I was working and earning good money. His brother's wife once told me, "Could not find any other men! This person is a cheat!." Then, I learned that he had been cheating on me all this while.

These revelations took a heavy toll on her mental well-being and eventually precipitated the onset of an SMI. Even after all these years, while recollecting those initial phases of the illness, Lavanya gained clarity by assigning meaning to it through her existing belief system. She believed that the illness was a consequence of the black magic done by her husband. She read materials on black magic, which further substantiated her belief.

> I became ill soon after because of the black magic my husband did to me. But I stopped caring for myself, going to work, eating, and bathing. I read a book called The Art of Black Magic and Witchcraft. I knew it was all happening because of that.

She was admitted to the Institute of Mental Health (IMH) in Chennai and treated there for a month. When she started responding to the medication, she was discharged. However, her tiffs with her husband worsened after this. Previously an asset to him, her husband started considering her a burden because of her diagnosis. And, now that he could not exploit her financially since she lost her job due to her illness, he initiated using her parents by asking for dowry, a patriarchal ritual to which Lavanya did not bow.

> After I was released, I did not want to work. My husband was continuously blaming my family and me. He would say, "You are mental, your parents are mental, your whole family is mental!." Then, he started asking for money from my parents.

Moreover, the diagnosis made it challenging for her to remain "socially acceptable."

> We were living in rented houses. So, whenever the house owner came to know that I had been to IMH, he would either raise the rent or ask us to vacate the house. I was frustrated with all these. So, I left him and the home and returned to my parents.

Eventually, agonised with these dejections, Lavanya returned to her parents, who, though sheltered her, could not accept her back unconditionally. Instead, she faced criticism and judgement.

> My father constantly taunted me, saying, "I had asked you not to marry this guy; still, you did. Now see what has happened to you!." Neither my parents nor my husband took care of me. I had one best friend. But she stopped being in touch after I came back from IMH. She did not allow me back at her house. I lost all contact with her eventually.

The treatment was discontinued during this time, and amidst their criticisms, her primary caregivers overlooked that Lavanya was relapsing. And, in no time, during a manic episode, she ran away from home. She was admitted to the IMH by a community member and was reported missing by the police. However, the police could trace her back, and she returned to her parents after being discharged. But, the dynamics of all the familial relations had altered with her diagnosis and consecutive admissions to the hospital.

> After I was released, my parents, siblings, husband, and everybody would talk to me about being admitted to IMH. It was not very reassuring. It was as if I was a person only with mental illness but nothing else. So I left my husband and went to my parents. But there also, my father was continuously critical of me.

Overwhelmed with betrayal, Lavanya got a job and left home again to stay at a hostel.

> I got a job at a school as a warden and left home once I got that. Then I started working as the warden of a working women's hostel. After a few months, I left that job and joined another hostel. It was impossible to stay in the same position the moment they would know about my diagnosis.

Challenges to the Process of Recovery and Empowerment

In the subsequent years, Lavanya had on her resume the experience of working in various sectors, sometimes as a warden, a librarian, or a stenographer. She had relapsed in between, but somehow, she survived. But every time she relapsed, she lost the job and had to start afresh once the symptoms subsided. Looking back, some of those memories had faded, and she could not recollect them vividly. But, for what it was worth, Lavanya knew that her life was a lonely battle, not for anyone else to fight. Thus, when one of her colleagues referred her to The Banyan, she grasped the opportunity to ensure a safe shelter for herself.

> I was referred by a colleague in one of the hostels I was working on. I did not come here for a job. I came here to find shelter. But now, I also work here. I am happier here. At least no one calls me that I am from IMH. But here, too, I do not get proper respect.

Lavanya acknowledged the help she received from The Banyan. However, she identified that she was still considered a patient, not someone who had worked with them for the last 20 years. To her, the stigma associated with the label of mental illness had the propensity to ruin the life of anyone once tagged. Furthermore, that labelling undermined all other qualities Lavanya believed she had beyond suffering from SMI.

Once labelled as "mental, " you cannot command the much respect you had before. No one should be labelled. The whole life gets spoilt. The chances of everything reducing. Everything is gone, and we live for the sake of living. I like the job, but they must recognise my skills and experience. I am not acknowledged for all these years of service.

There was a time in her life when Lavanya used to think of having an independent life without being identified as "mentally ill." For years, she found it difficult to remain hopeful of that future and to establish a separate identity beyond that label. She experienced betrayal, dejection, and denial from all possible familial, social, or systemic sources. Growing wiser with age and experiences, a septuagenarian Lavanya had developed her life's philosophy, "I do not think about what would happen later. I told you before, what you cannot cure, you have to endure, and I am doing that."

Muraad

Muraad was one of the three participants whom I interviewed at The Banyan's male shelter house in Chennai. His refined sophistication in his demeanour made him a contrast to his co-residents. It was one of those few interviews that I conducted in Chennai, where I did not require a translator because, all the while, Muraad conversed in fluent English.

Brought up in a well-to-do household, Muraad went to English-medium schools when it was still not the "trend" of every Indian home. At the age of 8, his father transferred to Kuwait. There too, he enjoyed a happy childhood and teenage years, becoming the captain of the school football team and graduating high school with flying colours. He recollected

Since we lived in an Indian community, the students at my school were Indian. I made new friends. I was good at my studies. I became a goalkeeper and the captain of my school football team. So I got a good reputation. I had a few girlfriends, also.

Life was idyllic for him till his father started deciding his career path, as is the norm in the "patriarchal society" in India. Muraad wanted to study aerospace engineering, while his father wanted him to be a doctor, and they moved back to India. Muraad felt demoralised, yet he chose to do his best with what he had.

It is one of the best medical colleges in the country. I did academically well. I also completed one independent research project. The college principal supervised me whenever I needed help. I was working on molecular memory. I received much appreciation from my professors. I was very popular among my friends.

However, he had also started consuming hashish during this time, which he claimed had no adverse effect on his academic performance. During the last six months of his medical training, life changed abruptly because of some unforeseen events, and he had still been looking for an explanation even after all these years.

Aspects of Social Suffering Associated with the Process of "Becoming" HMI Person Shaped by Familial and Socio-political Context

As Muraad recollected, he visited his parents in Allahabad just before start-ing his medical internship. He was very excited before this visit because he had been selected for his postgraduate degree in another prestigious Institute and could not wait to share the news with them. However, nothing could prepare him for a series of events and the following experiences.

> After completing the MBBS exams, I went home when I was just left with my internship. I told my father that I had passed my exams. I did not know what had happened. He slapped me and asked me to leave the house. I tried to defend myself. But he did not listen to me, and I had to leave the house. When my mother tried to stop him, he said she could follow me. I returned to my apartment near my college, but I did not want to return to college. Things were falling apart for me. I could not make sense of any of the things that were happening.

Feeling oppressed by this authoritarian attitude of his father, humiliated Muraad could not make any sense of the event. Thus, when his parents forced him to leave college and go and stay with his maternal grandparents in Allahabad, he complied. However, the feeling of alienation did not leave him there, and Muraad started getting stuck in the vicious cycle of substance intake and persistent low mood, both of which continued untreated.

> I was too upset and confused to do anything. There was a medical shop. I worked there for a few months. I did not have the money to buy my hashish. I was getting reckless. I took some medicines from the shop and had them. It made me go crazy. I was running on the streets with-out knowing what was happening.

Following that incident, he lost his shelter at his grandparents. He tried to contact his parents, but no amount of striving availed him. And it was during this period that he learned that he was not a biological child of his parents but adopted from his maternal aunt. Knowing this, Muraad sought shelter from his birth mother as his last resort.

> My biological father was long dead. So I went to my mother, who lived in an interior part of Allahabad with my younger sister and brother. My

mother took me to Agra, and I was put into the Asylum for quite some time. Then, finally, I got rid of the addiction.

Once out of the mental health hospital, he decided to complete his internship and went to Bangalore to pursue that. However, as a final nail to the coffin, the Institute denied him another chance. He could not make himself go back to Allahabad to his mother. He started staying on the streets and, thus, began his journey of being a homeless individual and surviving the plights.

Muraad attempted to gain some clarity about his symptoms and the suffering associated with them. He identified the cumulative effect of his stressful life events that culminated in his breakdown.

One after the other, it was too much to tolerate. Finally, I had a mental breakdown. I did not come back to Allahabad. I started living at the Bangalore railway station. I was crying all the time. I would assume the dogs were following me everywhere. I was trying to make sense of everything that was happening to me. I used to be very violent at times. I got stuck on the streets, and my parents did not want me. My biological mother did not wish me up and gave me up for adoption, and my adoptive parents did not wish me. I was running away from life.

All these years later, he could not even account for all he had lost to SMI.

Every student I knew, the good, the bad, the worst, all passed out and left. They got married, had children, and they have grown old. And for me, it is nothing. I got nothing. The mental breakdown took away everything.

Life on the streets, as he recollected, was harsh, "it was mainly surviving the extreme weather conditions, the rain, and the winter; life could not be any more problematic; there were many others like me around. In winter, I managed with a plastic blanket."

Though this harshness forced him to learn survival strategies, life did not become any more manageable. "Sometimes, I would beg for food. At times, the temples or food stalls give food. I slept on the platform. No one minded me being there. But it was never easy, not even for a day," he recalled. Finally, volunteers from a beggars' home rescued him in Bangalore, where he was treated for his SMI by a psychiatrist. He was discharged when he expressed his will to travel to Delhi to stay with his biological sister, who was married by then.

I came to Delhi after being released. My sister was married by then, and she was living in Delhi. I managed to reach her place. She let me stay with them. I stayed there for quite some time, but then my medication was discontinued, and I relapsed. I again became violent. They drove me out of their house.

On being denied the shelter, he had no option but to return to his life of homelessness; "I started living on the Delhi railway station platform. Again, the same lifestyle, the extreme weathers of Delhi made it even more difficult." Again, he was rescued by another NGO in Delhi while he suffered a heat-stroke, which sheltered him there. He requested that NGO send him to the "beggars' home" in Bangalore; from there, they sent him to The Banyan in Chennai. He had been staying there since 2014.

Challenges to the Process of Recovery and Empowerment

He identified that being rescued from the streets by the NGO saved his life. However, though he would appreciate staying independently outside the NGO, he felt a lack of confidence after all these years.

> I want to do that (living independently). I can arrange for some money, but how would I survive in the long run? I have no one to look after me, and I am getting old. I need people around.

Ageing and his lack of job experience kept him from taking any risk when it came to becoming financially empowered. Nevertheless, he also attributed it to his highly skilled training to become a doctor.

> I was building a medical career. Thus, any other job looks menial in comparison. I can either pursue a career in that or quit. I am not ready to do any menial tasks. I cannot do manual labour, and I cannot sell fruits on the streets. I cannot be a rickshaw puller. I would struggle to get back to my medical career. If not, then I quit. But anything other than that is not an option.

Because of staying disconnected from mainstream society for such a long time, Muraad found it difficult to relate. This also held him back from trying to push himself against the margin. And thus, when a friend offered him to live out of the NGO after all these years, he found himself unprepared.

> My friend came and took me to Kerala. But it was challenging to man-age life outside a shelter house. Our lives are very different. So, it was difficult for me to adjust there. It was a different place. I was not able to relate. And so, I came back.

Muraad has struggled with homelessness and SMI for over 30 years. However, not having adequate social support, a family or any meaningful, significant relationship made this struggle meaningless for him.

I had no choice but to fight, as I could not give up. Suicide is a crime. I survived because I had to. Nobody cares what I do. Sometimes I feel that this struggle would have been meaningful if anyone cared for me.

This same meaninglessness impeded him from moving beyond clinical recovery towards personal recovery and empowerment. Nevertheless, he chose to fight against all the odds that life put up across his way, survive homelessness, SMI, and never give up!

Nalini

Born to a lower-middle SES family, Nalini enjoyed her childhood despite some financial hiccups. The fond memories shared with her parents and siblings were more precious to her than attending an *expensive* school over a corporation school. She recollected having a solid bond with her cousin and aunt.

I was very close to my aunt, my father's sister. I would often go to visit her from school or work. I would go and have food at her place, sleep, and chat with her and my cousins. My aunt would comb my hair and make braids. I loved talking to her. I was like a daughter to her and closer to my cousins (sisters) than my sisters. We used to go to movies and beaches together.

Aspects of Social Suffering Associated with the Process of "Becoming" HMI Person Shaped by Familial and Socio-political Context

Academically not proficient, Nalini left school after the fourth standard when she could not get promoted after a couple of attempts. So she started helping her mother with household chores. But she was soon to experience life would not be a smooth journey for her being a woman in the male-dominant society when she got molested by her employer where she was the house help.

I was 17 years old. I was working as a house help. The person was respectable in society with grown-up kids who were doctors and engineers. One day I was sewing on the sewing machine, and he came and groped me from the back. I cursed him, saying, "Get leprosy and die." I stopped working at that place. I was of his granddaughter's age, and he did that to me! I felt disgusted.

She dealt with the situation with utmost dignity and firmness, but it shook her faith in the world's goodness. When Nalini turned 20, her parents, without any explanation, warned her that she should not think of getting married. The naïve girl did not dare to seek an answer from them then. Such were the norms. Thus, her parents were adamant when she fell in love and wanted to marry a colleague. They forced her to break up with the boy.

But I fell in love when I was 24 years old. I started working at a medical factory. I was to marry the chemist who worked there. However, my parents forced me to break up with him. He used to come to our house to meet me. My parents told him about my naga dosha, and he refused to marry me.

Overwhelmed with the feeling of being betrayed and dejected by her parents and the man she loved, heartbroken, Nalini tried to commit suicide. However, on getting discharged from the hospital, her parents told her about her having *naga dosha*, an astrological problem they believed she had.

I felt embarrassed because of that. My father did not tell me before that I had naga dosha, and I was a fool not to ask him why I was not allowed to marry. I only came to know that after I attempted suicide.

Nalini felt dehumanised and suffocated by being victimised by these cultural norms maintained by the patriarchal practices. Already clinically suffering from severe persistent low mood, this label of *naga dosha* added to her pain further. Furthermore, she became a victim of rumours from her friends and neighbours.

I got a bad name in society. I had told a friend about my love and suicide attempt; she told someone else, and soon everyone else knew about it. I used to be humiliated for it; they said I was probably pregnant, which is why I had attempted suicide!

Emotionally devastated by societal humiliation and personal losses, Nalini suffered a psychological breakdown. With a family history of SMI (her brother and a cousin were already diagnosed with SMI), Nalini was already vulnerable and prone to suffering from a SMI. The stressors catalysed and hastened the process.

Despite seeking treatment, some of her symptoms (mainly auditory hallucinations) stayed back. Furthermore, with the subsequent diagnosis of SMI in two of her sisters, it became impossible for the elderly parents to take care of them. Following the death of the brother and another sister, the helpless parents and another sibling thus decided to bring them under the continuous supervision provided by the NGO.

Even after being diagnosed with a mental illness, I continued working. But one time, the voices asked me to walk in the drain. I did what they said. My parents found it challenging to manage me at home. After that incident, they brought me here. On the other hand, my sister would often run away from home. That's why they got her here.

Nalini understood their helplessness despite missing her family members. Thus, even 18 years later, she found her meaning of home with her loved ones, not at the shelter -house.

Home brings joy. Home means I can be free, and I can do whatever I want to do. I can cook, go out, and go to the temple, and there are no restrictions. Home means living with family. This (the NGO) is not home. I do not have a home.

Challenges to the Process of Recovery and Empowerment

Nalini acknowledged the help she had received from the NGO over all these years. She felt grateful to them for providing her sister and her shelter and all the requirements for all these years. But her age and physical ailments posed further challenges on her way. Along with that, there were treatment-resistant auditory hallucinations.

I hear ten voices now. I would listen to them till I die, I guess! Seven voices say good things, and three say terrible things. There is one voice that helps me to sort things out and make decisions. It is the voice of that chemist whom I thought I would marry. But these other voices would say contradicting things and confuse me. They are in my head and would talk to me, even when I do not want to. Initially, I used to listen to their instruction, but now I do not listen to what they say.

Though she had acquired strategies to deal with the voices she heard over the years, they sometimes took a toll on her. Having no one to look after herself outside the NGO apart from her resourceless ailing parents and a widow sister, Nalini had no further expectations from her life. Moreover, having diabetes has reduced her working capabilities in the last couple of years.

Nalini had submitted all her sufferings to the all-mighty, praying only for strength to survive all that was still in the hold.

Lord Krishna is all I have. I pray to him; he provides me with strength. I pray to God that I should die soon. My health is not right; I have lived my life. I have no hope for the future. There is no way to a better life, and there is no reason. I have no one to care for, no husband or children. When you die, it is independence. Only death would bring me joy.

Considering that she had lived her share of life, Nalini, thus, awaited death, believing that it would bring along the joy and independence this life failed to offer her.

The purpose of the present chapter was to enunciate the life stories of those participants who got stuck at the barriers of social suffering they came across in their journeys of life. For Ruhi and Kavita, the myriad of abuses inflicted by the patriarchal power processes, the life as a "homeless" far from their homelands, along with the burden of SMI might have deprived them of those streaks of hopefulness that could have guided them further towards recovery and empowerment. Similarly, living in the latter halves of their lives, grappling with geriatric issues, and the suffering associated with homelessness and SMI, Lavanya, Muraad, and Nalini might have lost that zeal with which they started to persevere and challenge the odds. In all these five stories, the apparent absence of significant others or anything to look ahead to in their immediate future might have stripped them of the hope for "better days ahead." Their stories, thus, echoed their sole wish to live life as it had been at that moment (even though they were not content with it) after finding no meaning in their lifelong suffering.

In the following chapter, I would share some life stories where the individuals had started to push against the barriers of social suffering, homelessness, and SMI in their pathways of life. However, with overpowering reasons like their advancing age or the absence of significant others (as we also observed in this chapter), they lost the momentum to carry on that struggle. While they experienced contentment in their present status, we would see how due to the absence of "hope," they might have stopped garnering their vision towards some meaning or a more meaningful future.

Note

1 While Ruhi claimed her mother suffered with mental distress, it could not be clarified. However, there is sufficient evidence in literature to support a bidirectional relationship between domestic violence and mental distress (Trevillion et al., 2012; Sagar & Hans, 2018).

References

Bandyopadhyay, P. (2018, May 21). ফিরে এসেছে স্মৃতি, ঘরের পথে দুই বাংলাদেশি কন্যা. Anandabazar.com. Retrieved from https://www.anandabazar.com/state/west-bengal-news-police-recovered-two-mentally-ill-bangladeshi-girl-from-city-1.803062#.XzD2ZiIBUKs

Sagar, R., & Hans, G. (2018). Domestic violence and mental health. *Journal of Mental Health and Human Behaviour, 23*(1), 2.

Trevillion, K., Oram, S., Feder, G., & Howard, L. M. (2012). Experiences of domestic violence and mental disorders: A systematic review and meta-analysis. *PloS One, 7*(12), e51740.

4 Re-constructing the Withering Hopes

In the previous chapter, I illustrated the stories of those individuals who survived homelessness-SMI but lost their motivation to come out of that maze of suffering. In this chapter I would share a few life stories in which the individuals experience the process of recovery and empowerment to some extent. All these stories are threaded with their contentment in their present state. However, as they lacked hope (the critical driving force in one's life), they did not find any meaning to continue their struggle against the current (stigma or demands of social and relational worlds) to return to mainstream community life. For "Ayesha," "Karunai," and "Shankar," their advanced age and associated ailments rendered their hope for a future appear bleak. On the other hand, for "Bijon" and "Sujaya," having no significant familial or social relation came in their way of developing or nurturing hope towards a meaningful future.

Ayesha

I met Ayesha Bibi on 3 November 2016, in her neighbourhood, one of the most crowded areas of Kolkata, Rajabazar. I was comfortable in that area because of my two years of University in the same locality. I sat with her on the pavement beside her roadside shack. Gradually, as we talked, her neighbours started gathering around us. It recreated the inquisitive neighbourhood feeling that lies core to the spirit of Kolkata. This "over inquisitiveness of the neighbours" had been one of the critical factors that gave Iswar Sankalpa the courage to start their outreach programme "Naya Daur." The community in Kolkata has always been interested in discovering what's happening to the person next to it. This makes the community engage with everything around, from football to tea-stall *adda* (gatherings), to politics, to taking care of the dishevelled *pagal* (mad person) in the locality. That is how I heard Ayesha's story, partly from her and partly from her neighbours who had witnessed her suffering and growth.

DOI: 10.4324/9781032662053-4

Aspects of Social Suffering Associated with the Process of "Becoming"
HMI Person Shaped by Familial and Socio-political Context

Ayesha's experience of being dehumanised by the patriarchal power process started as a child. Like most girls, it started at home. She recollected being physically abused by her stepmother, but the emotional humiliation she experienced was much more deep-seated.

> My parents were very aggressive. My mother had two "*nikah*" (marriages); my father also did the same. No one took care of me. I used to cry for food; the stepmother would beat me. She would beat me till I became senseless. I was hardly five years, and I would roam around in the neighbourhood.

She could understand her father's helplessness. He used to ask her to get herself out of that place, "My father used to feel bad for me. He asked me to go away from there to save myself, and so I came to Kolkata with my aunt."

Hoping to have a better life, Ayesha started living with her aunt on the pavements of Kolkata and working as a child labour. After a year or two, Ayesha's mother joined her there.

> Her (mother's) second husband was dead, and so was my father. So she came to Kolkata and made a shack on the footpath at that corner (she pointed her finger towards one edge of the pavement on the opposite side of the road). So I started living with her there. She found herself working as a labour, and she made me work with her.

But the poverty continued, "I used to beg the bread as I did before. She (her mother) would boil it in the water, and we would have it with some sugar." After coming to Kolkata, within two years, Ayesha's mother got her married off to a fellow pavement-dweller. Ayesha's exploitation because of the patriarchal practices and her helpless struggle against poverty continued.

> I was ten when my mother got me married. After that, I started living with my husband. But even there, I had to struggle to make ends meet. He would bring one Kg of rice and say it's two Kgs. I was beaten like anything by him. But he has been dead for fifteen years now.

Ayesha's experience with homelessness began as early as she was five. It continued till the last day of her life. However, during the later phase, she could build a shack for herself that she considered home. She recollected her childhood days of surviving homelessness before marriage.

> I would beg in the neighbourhood. People would give me one or a half roti (bread). That used to be enough for me. I bathed in the street taps, slept on the roadside verandas, and fed myself on that half piece of roti.

Ayesha could not remember exactly when her mental illness started but it was after a few years of her husband's death. He could recollect fragments of her suffering during that phase.

> I used to roam around the streets, rag-picking and abusing people, spitting or shouting at them. People used to hate me. No one looked after me, my daughter, her husband, or my neighbours.

Unable to find any meaning to her lifelong misery, poverty, homelessness, and, above all, the SMI, bewildered helpless Ayesha would question the All-Mighty, trying to gain clarity through her existing belief system.

> I often think about what I have done so wrong that I am suffering throughout life! I used to cry and pray to Allah. What have I done? No one looked after me, my mother, father, husband or children! You are the Supreme who can do anything! Why do You not help me?

Ayesha recounted feeling betrayed and dejected about being denied shelter and treatment even by her children, for whom she had struggled all her life.

> They were little. I worked a day in and out. My sons worked as well. (I) got them all married. My sons have left with their wives. I got my daughter married. (I) gave her husband ten thousand rupees to make a shack of their own, but then they took over my shed also.

Process of Recovery and Empowerment

Ayesha identified that her life started improving after getting treatment for her mental illness. She acknowledged Iswar Sankalpa for that, "It was then when the "dada" (addressing social worker as a brother) found me. The doctor gave me medicines. I did not have them initially, but then I started to have the medication."

She further talked about how the community members played a critical role in her treatment because she was not taken to the NGO shelter-house but treated as part of the outreach programme of Iswar Sankalpa. In the initial phase, a proxy caregiver was assigned from the community to take care of her medicine. Later, once her active symptoms subsided, and she was on maintenance treatment, Ayesha took responsibility for her medications.

While the NGO made accessibility to resources viable, Ayesha remained in the driver's seat in this new phase of her life. First, she found a job at a roadside eatery. After that, she started getting satisfaction and meaning in her current empowered status, where she was loved, respected, and cared for in the community.

> They love me a lot at my workplace. They ask me to bring tea or cigarette for them. The owner would shout at the other employees for

bothering me like that. I am happy now. I don't have any problems or pain now. My neighbours also take care of me. They all love me.

But Ayesha did not feel motivated to outgrow what she had at present. With whatever little she had been earning, she was content. At this time, I had to stop my interview since Ayesha suddenly started having a seizure episode. On asking, I learned that Ayesha had been having such episodes for the last week. It had gone unidentified by the social worker for the last week as she did not mention it to him. The episodes apparently started after she stopped her medicine all of a sudden as she believed it was causing frequent micturition.

What would I do with any more money? I have lived all my life on these pavements. And now, I am at the edge of it. I have nothing but to wait for death to come. I don't hope for anything from anyone. I am done!

He was having trouble at her workplace because of excusing herself frequently. So she stopped the medication without consulting or informing anyone. Since then, she has had these episodes where her neck would turn to a side, and her mouth would tighten to that side, with drooling and altered consciousness lasting for 20–40 seconds (a partial seizure with secondary generalisation due to Olanzapine withdrawal). The frequency of the episodes had increased from one or two on the first day to six to seven times over the next few days.

I was clueless about what I should do at that moment. After Ayesha gained consciousness, I tried to gather the required information for a medical treatment to follow. I asked the social worker to immediately contact his coordinator and take Ayesha Bibi to the Neurology Department of a nearby Government Medical College (walking distance from where she stayed). She had two more episodes within 30 minutes as we tried to coordinate things. Finally, the social worker took her to the hospital. I came back home.

I called the social worker that night to find out what the doctor said. But my call went unreceived. Due to some reasons, I could not go to the field the next day. I met the social worker on Saturday as I entered the Shelter-house. He looked devastated! I stopped to ask him about Ayesha Bibi. What he said was beyond my comprehension! Beyond my logical reasoning! That day he had taken her to the Neurology department. They asked to get an MRI done. But many people were waiting before her. It was already late afternoon. They thought they would come back the next morning. The following day, even before he could reach, Ayesha Bibi was rushed to the hospital by her neighbours and declared brought dead owing to a severe cardiac arrest.

I initially decided not to transcribe this narrative. I was scared to revisit the life story of Ayesha Bibi. Her life story was not much different from the stories I had collected across Kolkata's streets. Its pages were yet again filled with her days and nights of extreme physical abuse since childhood, lifelong poverty, the perpetual struggle against the current to reach the mainstream society and sustain there, nothing new, nothing exceptional. However, what happened during the interview and the next couple of days, once again made me stand face to face with that eternal question – How transient is life? And it made me realize that I need to find a place to tell Ayesha's story in her own voice. This is my homage to Ayesha, acknowledging her lifelong suffering, which she endured with zeal even though we, the stakeholders and society, failed her at so many levels.

Karunai

Karunai was one of the few participants I could interview across the two phases of my fieldwork at Chennai. Though the follow-up interview happened almost four months later, she could remember me from our first meeting. A woman in her late sixties with a jovial smile on her lips, her features reminded me of an adorable grandmother. Even when I had not interviewed her, she would greet me warmly whenever I went for a coffee at the café she worked. Thus, when I approached her for the interview, she readily agreed to share her life story.

Aspects of Social Suffering Associated with the Process of "Becoming"
HMI Person Shaped by Familial and Socio-political Context

Born to a family of lower-socio-economic background, Karunai had been struggling against poverty all her life. The fifth born of eight siblings, she had to quit schooling after the seventh standard. Karunai recollected the everlasting financial crisis.

> My parents had to buy books and pay the school fees as well. How could they afford it? So, I left. There were goats near my house, a neighbour's. I used to take them to the field for grazing. I got paid for that. All the other siblings worked as well.

Though she had to leave school due to a lack of money, she was okay with it. Primarily for two reasons: first of all, she had no cash or other options that would provide for her education. She commented, "Now the government offers books, payments, and free food. But before, it was not there." Second, in a rural setup in Tamil Nadu four to five decades ago, it was not uncommon for kids, let alone girls, to quit studying before finishing school. Thus, even though she liked it when she went to school, she did not mind leaving it either since everyone around her was doing the same. Succumbing to the patriarchal power processes and adjusting to them by normalising them, Karunai soon learnt to concentrate on household chores.

When Karunai was in her late teens, she stayed with her pregnant sister to care for her. Soon after that, her brother-in-law asked her hand for marriage, which Karunai found intensely offensive and humiliating. Infuriated, she firmly refused, and her parents stood by her. However, the brother-in-law felt insulted because of this rejection and retaliated by abusing her sister physically and emotionally.

In their family, everyone had two marriages. It was a custom for them. It became a prestige issue when I said no. He started torturing my sister so that I would say yes. (My sister) came to me and asked me to marry him and have a child. They already had five children of their own. But then he used to torture her physically because I refused to marry him.

When the situation went out of her parents' control, they complained to the police to save their daughters' fates. But the brother-in-law left the town with her sister and their children, detaching all contact. This was a source of agony for the entire family, especially Karunai, who felt responsible for the distress the incident caused her parents. It took a toll on her mental well-being; she identified this as a stressor precipitating the mental illness.

All these, my sister being tortured, her asking me to marry him, the police involvement, these were all very upsetting. I became heartbroken after this. I don't know what happened. One day I left home with a Bible and a Quran and went to my brother's place. I was shouting and abusing people verbally. My brother had to slap me to calm me down. The mental problems started from there.

Her caregivers' lack of awareness about mental health conditions intensified her suffering. Instead of considering medical help, she was taken to the mosque. However, at the suggestion of the *maulabi* (the priest), she was admitted to the hospital. Karunai remembered being cared for dearly by her relatives during this time.

When I was in the hospital, my mother or my sister-in-law (brother's wife) would be there to take care of me. I was given medicines to sleep through the day and night. My family brought me home and gave me the medication regularly. After that, I was eating and sleeping. I don't remember most things but what my family told me when I was doing better.

As she started responding to the medicines clinically, her parents decided to get her married and sought an alliance for her. However, this was done without consulting her treating doctor. Though the in-laws were informed about her diagnosis of a mental health condition, Karunai discontinued her medicines soon after the wedding. Though she did not reflect on why she did that, it might be because of the intense stigma associated with her diagnosis and taking medication for it. However, on relapse, she was put on medication again.

Karunai shared a good relationship with her in-laws, particularly her mother-in-law. However, the relationship with the husband had been strained from the beginning, mainly because of his drinking and anger management issues.

He used to get very angry if I talked to others, especially men. He would shout at me then and misunderstand me. He often told me I was very fat and looked like my mother. To his mother, he would say that she brought me home and that she should take care of me as he was not interested in me.

These occasional tiffs turned into regular fights when they moved out of the joint family 15 years later and shifted to another town due to her husband's transfer. She would often relapse during this time. As a result, she left her children (a daughter and a son) with her in-laws. However, no one consulted her when her daughter's marriage was fixed. As a result, she felt humiliated and dejected. Outraged, Karunai left home to stay at a shelter house. But she was sent back home because she had no identity proof. Still angry with her husband and in-laws, she went to visit her brother but soon relapsed as she was off medication again.

I would become angry without any reason, not doing anything, shouting at everybody. My family members did not like that. Finally, my brothers' wives would allow me to stay for a month, but because of my behaviour, they sent me back to stay with my husband. But my husband was never interested in me. We were always fighting, and I again came out of the home. I don't remember what happened this time. But I was later told I was roaming the streets, abusing people. One of the madams saw me there, and she brought me here in an auto.

Though Karunai recalled that she had left home whenever she relapsed, she would most of the time be in the neighbourhood. She could be traced back home, except for this time. The apathy of her husband and other family members against her symptoms, the lack of treatment adherence over the years, and definite negligence on the part of the service providers jeopardised her life further when she ended up on the streets.

On being rescued from the streets, she was treated at the female shelter house of The Banyan. A few months later, she could recall her brother's details. But, when the NGO tried to contact them, her sister-in-law refused shelter.

One person from The Banyan went to my home. My brother's wife, my sister-in-law, shouted at him, saying she would not let me stay with them and they would no longer take any responsibility for me.

Karunai started living at The Banyan's shelter house. Soon, she started participating actively in regular chores. Seeing her spontaneity, she was employed as a cook in the café that the residents run at the shelter-house premise. A year later, getting to know her whereabouts from her brother, Karunai's husband came to fetch her from the shelter house. But at home, due to a lack of supervision and appropriate care, Karunai discontinued her medication once more and relapsed. She came out of the house again and ended up at the shelter house by sheer chance. She responded to the medicines soon enough and chose not to return home because of all the negative experiences accumulated over the years.

> I don't want to. The caregivers say I should go back because I am doing well, but I don't want to. I have run away from home many times. When I returned, people considered me not a good character because I ran away, and they talked about me. The last time I went home, my younger brother's wife told me, "You stay in the shelter house; no good woman stays there. We are already taking care of your children, and we are not going to take care of you".

Despite having the choice of going home again, Karunai chose to stay at the shelter-house because back in the mainstream, she felt alienated and marginalised mainly because of the stigmatised identity of being a "woman who has SMI and who had been homeless." It further exacerbated the feeling of being a "burden to her caregivers."

> My mother depended on my brothers; though she cared about me, she would tell me to go to my husband's because my brothers would not look after me. The last time I went home, my husband had been very caring. He had been asking me to rest and do the chores. But after all these years of fighting, I felt like I am a burden on him. So, I should stay here.

Her sense of being betrayed by the caregivers on being denied care and treatment created a sense of loss suffered by SMI. Furthermore, it also reshaped her meaning of home.

> I feel homeless when I am with my husband or other family members. A home is a place where you need not be alone. I feel lonely there. Instead, I like being here. The shelter is my home. I like that there are so many people here. They want to send me to a group home. There will be other people along with me. I feel okay when there are people around me.

The loss further rendered her guilty as a mother who had failed her children.

> I miss my children. My children were reared by their paternal aunts and grandmother. Because I used to come out of the house whenever I was angry, leaving my kids behind, they were concerned about their (children's) safety. So, I don't have a close relationship with either of them.

I failed them. I could not take care of any of my responsibilities because of my illness. I could not take care of my children as a mother. I could not take care of myself, let alone others!

Process of Recovery and Empowerment

Karunai did not regret her decision to stay back at The Banyan. On the contrary, she perceived the NGO as a parent, providing her with all the necessary resources and accepting her unconditionally even when blood relations failed her.

> The Banyan has been like a parent to me. They have never asked me to leave. When I used to go to my parents, people would ask me to go to my husband. When I went there, they would ask me to go to my parents. For me, everyone faced problems. So, I would rather be here than with them.

The chosen pathway to homelessness redefined home for her, as mentioned earlier. Within the limited range of the shelter-house, she had once again found a way to develop social support for herself based on mutual understanding and empathy.

> I am here with everyone else. The NGO gave me food, clothes, and a place to sleep. I have got my friends here. I talk about my past with them and take care of each other; it feels good, like being at home.

Challenges to the Process of Recovery and Empowerment

Despite overcoming numerous hurdles, a few challenges posed on the way have slowed Karunai down from seeking a future beyond her clinical recovery and contentment with the necessities being provided.

> I think nothing about my future. I am working here, getting some money at the end of the month. I am okay with whatever the NGO decide for me. You people think a lot. With you, it is different. But I don't think so much. I go to the kitchen, and I work there. I don't think about the past. I don't want to think about how life would have been different. I don't know if my life has been affected or not. I used to listen to whatever the voices used to say; when they asked me to leave home, I used to do that. I never really thought.

Having been betrayed various stages of her life, she found herself with nothing to hope for in particular. Moreover, based on her past experiences, she also apprehended being stigmatised if she tried to explore her life out in the world. Besides that, her difficulty maintaining treatment adherence when unsupervised also made it more difficult for her to rely entirely on herself for self-sustenance. Furthermore, inadequate exposure to the outside world, her increasing age and associated ailments, and her lack of any definitive goal in her immediacy rendered her hope for the future appear bleak.

Shankar

My interaction with Shankar happened at a roadside tea stall which belonged to his proxy caregiver. Living there for all these years had made him "Shankar da" to all the other stall owners and regular customers. While we talked, they joined the conversation on and off while we talked, adding their experiences with Shankar over the years. It also helped me to picture how Shankar became a part of mainstream society with community help and cooperation.

Aspects of Social Suffering Associated with the Process of "Becoming" HMI Person Shaped by Familial and Socio-political Context

Shankar's share of suffering started early in life with the premature death of his father. From what he could remember, his father had also suffered mental illness. Before that, life was good because his father earned well. But when he fell ill, there was no turning back from that.

> My father had died early. He had also become pagal (mad). He used to go away from the house at times. Finally, he had to be admitted to a hospital. There was no financial crisis when he was alive. He worked in a big company. He got my sisters married into well-to-do families, but none looked after him when he fell sick.

Shankar felt all his siblings betrayed his parents since neither of them looked after the parents. And even his mother died untreated. He recalled, "After my father's death, two years later, my mother became blind. I was ten years old then. When she died, there was no one to look after me. I was fifteen!"

Orphaned at 15, he was abused, threatened, and denied his right to property at home.

> They have physically abused me, also. Whenever I went home, they insulted me and shouted at me. All are evil. My brother loves me, but his wife, daughter, and son-in-law are cruel. They are jealous of me. They do not want to give me a share of my property. They wanted to have it all. My brother forced me to sign the will and give my share to him.

With his social networking skills, young Shankar arranged a job for himself. That job was enough to take care of his basic needs, "I knew someone in the bus union. He arranged work for me as a helper. I worked as a helper all my life until 10-12 years ago."

Feeling betrayed by his siblings, Shankar left home and started living on the streets, "I started living on the streets. Whenever I went home, they would abuse me and shout at me. I thought it is better to be on the roads." Even when homeless and suffering from mental illness, he continued his job. Shankar maintained this newly established status quo until he met with a fateful accident.

> I fell from the bus and was run over by a taxi. I was already suffering from mental illness then. I had a severe fracture in my hand and leg. I was admitted to the hospital for many days, probably months.

Though his family learned about him, no one visited him at the hospital. Neither took him home when discharged. However, once he got back from the hospital, the community members where he stayed on the street volunteered to look after him.

> The owners of these roadside food stalls all looked after me. "Sanju" (proxy caregiver) and his aunt would wash my wounds, take me for a check-up, buy my medicines, and give me food. They made a bed for me here.

While he received the help of the community, on the one hand, homelessness had negative consequences. He experienced dehumanisation and humiliation by being harassed physically and emotionally by some apathetic community members.

> Some boys throw water at me and call me names. I get furious when they do all this. I shout at them, throw stones, and abuse them. One time, I went to shave my beard, and they threw water on me. I got so angry that I smashed the mirror. Another time, a few boys were irritating me. I threw stones at them, and they cracked the glass of a car standing on the road. The owner came and took me inside the car and beat me severely. People had also stolen the money I had saved. I had them in my pocket, but they stole them while I was sleeping.

Shankar was unable to recollect when he started suffering from mental illness. But it was after his mother's death, followed by the abuses. "Mother's brother's." Then, while his memory had faded, he heard stories about his symptomatic days from the community members, which gave him some clarity.

> They (the community caregivers) tell me that I used to be talking and smiling to myself. I would stand in the middle of the road, controlling traffic. I could not take care of myself and would not bathe or wash my clothes.

Process of Recovery and Empowerment

Throughout the interview, Shankar talked about the facilitative roles Iswar Sankalpa and the community played by providing him accessibility to essential resources, "He (proxy- caregiver) takes care of everything about me, my food, clothes, medicine. All the other shopkeepers are also very helpful."

This unconditional acceptance that he received from them added meaning to his present. He experienced satisfaction and contentment with his improved quality of life. He felt socially resourceful and relevant in the newly developed social relations, especially with his proxy caregiver. On the other hand, he felt his blood relations had betrayed him. So, he did not look forward to going back to them. But the new ties that he had kindled were mutually dependent. It gave him a new meaning against all the past betrayals he had experienced all his life.

> He is my brother [his eyes twinkle as he talks about Sanju]. I am staying with him now. It feels like home. Every night we go back home together after closing the stall. On the way, we stop at times to buy things. Then we watch tv for some time. After that, he cooks dinner and serves us. I manage the shop all by myself when he goes out. I sleep at the stall at night when he is not in Kolkata.

While the newly developed relations gave him meaning for the present, his future still looked bleak and blurred, with no one to look forward to.

> My mother became blind in her last days. I would also get blind. My mother is gone, and my father is gone. I would go to them now. I have nothing in life anymore. I would live as long as I do not die [he sighs as tears roll down his wrinkled cheeks].

Along with that, his advanced age, lack of purpose, and any need to be financially self-sufficient posed as constraints that stagnated his journey towards recovery and empowerment after a point.

Bijon

I met Bijon across that bridge in Kolkata, where Iswar Sankalpa's outreach worker first identified him. Since he could not recall his name then, the NGO named them after the bridge for the time being. A few years down the lane, ironically, he was more comfortable in this new name than the one that carried the memories of the atrocities of his past life. As with Shankar, during my conversation with Bijon, the community members pitched in. It reflects how rehabilitation in the outreach helped sensitise the community about mental illnesses and their acceptance to a large extent.

Aspects of Social Suffering Associated with the Process of "Becoming"
HMI Person Shaped by Familial and Socio-political Context

His maternal grandparents brought up Bijon after the death of his parents. He could not recollect much about his parents and wanted to forget his childhood. Perceiving himself as a burden to his relatives, Bijon tried with all his might to meet their expectations. Still, the abuses he received made him realise he failed: "My uncle always abused me because I was of no good! Who would want to have someone of no use at home [sighs!]"? Despite that, Bijon adjusted to all the suffering associated with the relational processes; however, things got out of hand when he lost the job his uncle had found for him.

> My uncle found a job for me in a shoe box factory. I had to make the boxes there. But I was not good at it. So, I lost my job. One time I had to carry fifty boxes on my head from one place to another. But while taking them, some of the boxes fell into the puddle and got wasted. They started abusing me. I got angry, and I beat them back. They sacked me after that. My uncle got very angry with me and drove me out of the house!

The loss of the job, followed by the forced homelessness, reaffirmed in him his "uselessness," as his uncle claimed. Having nowhere else to go, Bijon started living on the streets of his neighbourhood. However, being denied his right to care and shelter, betrayed and dejected, even now, Bijon refuses to go back home to his relatives. His past experiences of abuse intimidated him and reshaped his meaning of home forever.

> I don't want to go back to my relatives. If I went to stay with them, they would again abuse me. When I was a child, they cared for me a lot. But now, things are different. I am now scared of my uncles.

It was unclear from his narrative when and how the mental illness started, but it was after becoming homeless. He could remember glimpses of his life as an HMI individual, experiencing the apathy of the community members and the police.

> (One day) I was standing near the Narkeldanga Bridge, all naked. The police came and told me that I would have to go with them. The local people started telling the police that they should take me away from that place. I have been a nuisance in the locality, standing in front of the tea stall all day, asking customers to buy me a cup. The police told me, "See, we are asking you respectfully come with us. We will take you to a place where you can stay and get food". I said I would not go. They said they would have to bring me in forcefully if I refused. They took me to a place and gave me food. But the next day, they said I should

leave, gave me 50 rupees, and made me go. After that, I used to roam the streets and ended up being here.

Misguided by the stakeholders, Bijon got displaced from the neighbourhood to which he was at the least accustomed. Surviving in the unknown streets of the city became more difficult.

One time, a taxi driver accused me of stealing his money. Then he went to the police station and complained about me. I told them many times that I did not take it. What would I do with the money? But they did not listen to me and put me in jail. Then "dada" (addressing proxy-caregiver as a brother) went there in the morning and got me released.

Process of Recovery and Empowerment

The outreach social worker identified him here, under the bridge. Once medically diagnosed with SMI by the psychiatrist of the NGO, the social worker next sensitised some community members and managed to create a proxy caregiver for Bijon. This proxy caregiver was a local shopkeeper, and he was responsible for giving Bijon his daily doses of medicines and food as and when provided by the social worker.

This "*dada*" (addressing a social worker from the NGO as a brother) found me under the bridge. I used to come to this shop (of the proxy caregiver) to ask for water. He always gave me water and food at times. Then this *dada* used to come to provide me with food and clothes. He made me take a bath, cut my hair, and shave. I have gradually become better. They gave me medicine. Now, I take my medication regularly. [smiles contently]

This unconditional acceptance from the NGO and the community gave Bijon that contentment in his life that he had never found before. Experiencing a relatively better quality of life, Bijon found himself resourceful to society in gaining back his functionalities.

I am staying in this shop. I open the shop and arrange it before he (the proxy caregiver) comes. I close it at night. I bring lunch to him from his house every day. I also run errands for other shopkeepers. For example, I carry ice for that shopkeeper who sells lime soda. They give me 10-20 rupees.

Though menial, Bijon enjoyed the errands he ran for the shopkeepers. It gave him the purpose of contributing to others' lives.

Challenges to the Process of Recovery and Empowerment

Even though he had been living a productive life and contributive life, the lack of hope in his immediate future had negatively catalysed Bijon's need to explore his self-sufficiency and empowerment further.

> What would I do with the money? I don't have anyone dependent on me. I get good food, clothes and a place to sleep. Everyone asks me to go and find a job and settle down. But I am fine here!

Furthermore, the lack of confidence he bore from the consistent dejections experienced all his life stopped him from aiming for something better for himself or dreaming of a better future.

> What work can I do? I am a mad person, and no one would trust me with any task. I am not capable of any such job. No one would marry someone like me, so I would never have a family.

Thus, having no significant source of hope, Bijon left all his worries to the all-mighty to take care of, "About the future, only *Khuda* knows. I have no plans. What will happen in the future is all up to Allah"!

Sujaya

I met Sujaya at the female shelter house "Sarbari" during the third phase of my fieldwork in Kolkata. It was in August 2017. I often observed this soft-spoken woman in her late thirties strolling in the hallway or the garden when not working. I approached her for an interview, and she readily agreed. It seemed she had a lot to say. So we sat for it on a lazy monsoon afternoon, cross-legged, on the floor of their classroom. It was raining cats and dogs that day, and I was in no hurry to go anywhere. We talked for three hours; she told me her story, and I shared my bits.

Sujaya was the only child born to her parents. Despite that, her mother gave her to be brought up by her maternal grandmother. Her father consented. She always knew that her mother had refused to take care of all her needs "to feed me, bathe me, dress me, everything that a child needs to be taken care of." However, she learned to find solace in the care she received from her grandmother and the occasional visits she had from her mother. The feeling of abandonment had been with her ever since. Adding to her void further, her mother passed away when she was just ten years. Remembering her, Sujaya recollected, "After she died, I thought I would not be able to ask anyone about her. She was wonderful. Tall and slim. I am not like her."

*Aspects of Social Suffering Associated with the Process of "Becoming"
HMI Person Shaped by Familial and Socio-political Context*

Sujaya's suffering seemed to have started with her mother's abandonment in infancy. Her mother's death in her childhood might have added to that manifold, especially when Sujaya was diagnosed with SMI in her teenage. It all started after an accident in which she suffered some burning. The injuries were more emotional than physical.

> I got burnt. My aunt was cooking. Sitting beside her, she was putting vegetables in the hot oil, and some hot oils got sprinkled on my cheek. I got scared that the wounds would never heal; the blisters would stay like that. I had a high fever. I feared that ghosts would harm me.

Once the injuries subsided and the fever was gone, she was taken to a faith healer as a primary treatment course because she was still afraid of "ghosts harming her." Sujaya tried to make sense of what was happening to her through her existing belief system and the precursor incidents. The faith healer's declaration reaffirmed it, "I was told it happens when someone is possessed by an evil spirit/ghost or when someone has done black magic using the menstrual cloth or blood."

Her distress and suffering associated with the symptoms persisted due to inadequate awareness about SMI among the caregivers. The symptoms exacerbated, going beyond the control of her caregivers, and she started wandering away from home; treatment from a general physician was sought. He referred them to a psychiatrist. With treatment, she started faring well. But because of the episodic nature of her illness, she would relapse at times.

With a diagnosis of mental health condition came the consequence of being labelled. Sujaya started feeling dejected and humiliated by experiencing social alienation at school, neighbourhood, and among her relatives.

> I had to leave school because of this. I used to have episodes at school. Neighbours and other relatives used to tell my uncle, "How can you keep her at home! She has mental problems! Send her to a hospital!". Later even my uncle used to say so. They used to keep me sedated all the time. I felt so helpless! I used to feel like I was no person. I am a liability to my uncle and the world!

Marriage is widely considered a solution to many problems within the socio-cultural framework of Indian patriarchal practices. And thus, she got married off. However, her in-laws were adequately aware of Sujaya's mental health condition, and treatment continued after marriage. Seeking the faith healer's help continued alongside.

> I had medicines. When I had the medication, I felt better. But I would be ill some other time. So my family would bring a tantric (faith healer) to perform some rituals on me at home. He used to give me amulets to wear.

The brunt of mental illness did not just stop with social alienation. After one year of marriage, Sujaya gave birth to a girl child. She continued relapsing episodically. Her mother-in-law, her pillar of support, was not keeping well. The financial condition of the family was also not good. Thus, they put the child in an orphanage.

> She (mother-in-law) said that I would not be able to take care of my child. I was not well most of the time. My mother-in-law was too ill. She said my daughter would be neglected in the family if something happened to her or me. So it's for her good that we sent her to the hostel. My mother-in-law passed away soon after that.

Sujaya persuaded herself that it was for the child's best. However, she could understand that she had lost her "experience of motherhood" to SMI.

Following the death of her mother-in-law, Sujaya's husband stopped taking her to the hospital.

> My husband stopped taking me to the hospital. I became more ill. I used to come out of the house and wander off. Initially, he used to bring me back home. Then he stopped doing that. I started living on the streets. I would sleep under the Dhakuria bridge or on the Dhakuria station platform.

In hindsight, Sujaya felt immensely betrayed by her husband for giving up on her and denying her rights to treatment, care, and shelter.

> He used to come and visit me at times. He used to give me some money and sometimes buy me some food. My aunt visited at times. Everyone knew where I was staying. Nevertheless, no one took me to the doctor or home. Then one day, my husband told me he had married again. He said he would not be able to look after me anymore.
>
> Sujaya futilely lamented the loss of everything she ever had to SMI.
>
> I got married into a good family, and they were good people. I used to tell everything to my mother-in-law. We went to the grocery shops together. We used to sit and talk, plant spinach in our garden, do other household chores, cook, and go to the vegetable market. It kept me distracted from my illness. I could have lived with my husband and daughter [eyes well up]. It could have spared all the expenditures that my treatment had incurred. I could have done my family's household chores and taken care of them. My daughter would have still lived with me. But I failed. I lost them, and I lost everything I ever had.

Soon after this, her husband passed away. Her grandmother had died much before that. Now, even her uncle refused her shelter or treatment.

He (uncle) was the only bread winner of the family. Above that, he had borne my treatment costs for a psychiatrist since I was eighteen. Then, when I got married, I became my husband's responsibility. So, when my husband also gave up, my uncle did not want to take care of me again.

And thus, there was no going back from the homeless life she was already living.

Sujaya reminisced about the tormenting life she had suffered and survived on the streets, the feeling of dehumanisation on being violated on multiple occasions for being vulnerable as a homeless person, particularly a woman.

Everyone looks down upon you when they know you are homeless and *pagol* (mad). Even the police raped me. One time I was sleeping on the platform; the policeman who was supposed to protect me took advantage of me. I pleaded to him, "Don't do this. My husband has asked me to stay here, don't do". He did not listen.

Sujaya had known life within a home where family meant everything. The consequent deaths of her primary caregivers (especially her grandmother and mother-in-law) rendered her homeless. At the same time, the other relatives refused her shelter at a later stage.

Nevertheless, her pathway to homelessness had been followed by her suffering SMI. She thus still believed that had there been no mental illness, she would not have lost her family or home. Therefore, her meaning of home was deeply enrooted in having a family where one would be mutually cared for.

This (NGO shelter-house) is no home. I have no one to love me here. It's an enclosed place. You have to live within the four walls (*bodhho jayega*). Home is where you do your work on your own, take care of your loved ones, and be with them.

Challenges to the Process of Recovery and Empowerment

Despite being unable to consider the shelter house a home, Sujaya could not think of having a shelter for herself outside its boundaries. She found it difficult to rebuild trust in others outside her social group. Hence, living outside independently appeared more challenging, mainly because she considered herself "vulnerable" as a woman.

I would stay here for the rest of my life. Where else can I go? The doctor is coming here. I can tell him whatever problems I have. Who else can I say? I have no money! My husband is dead. Now, I don't want to go out. People take advantage when they know that you are alone. My uncle and aunt are also not interested in having me over.

Though she recognised the importance of the safety and security provided by the NGO, she could not help but voice her concern about feeling unheard within the hierarchy of the setup.

> I'm not particularly eager to cook. They (caregivers at the shelter house) ask me to prepare food. I get burnt while cooking. I can do other jobs like bathing the old residents who cannot care for themselves. I am scared of going near the fire but not cooking. They don't understand that.

Process of Recovery and Empowerment

Sujaya expressed feeling secure about being rescued from homelessness by the NGO. She acknowledged them for providing access to essential resources. She expressed her satisfaction with her current status on regaining her functionality with improved life quality: "I never thought that I would be better. I would be able to study again, giving an exam. I also cut the vegetables, wash the fish." Losing all ties with her past life, Sujaya had been attempting to re-develop her social network based on empathy and mutual understanding with her fellow residents.

> I talk to people, yet I only have a few friends. But I feel happy to speak with Lakshmi. She has a good heart, like a child. I also try to talk to these girls, but they don't say anything. They don't say where they are from, their address, or anything. I feel so bad for them.

Sujaya had been trying to provide support socially and emotionally by attempting to recreate a new network. But the emptiness her past had rendered posed a challenge to the empowerment process. Sujaya could find no meaning in becoming self-sufficient and self-dependent or undertaking any endeavours to empower herself. This could be because of multiple reasons. All her life, Sujaya, like most other lower-middle-class women, had been financially dependent on her primary caregivers all her life. So much so that their deaths left her homeless without access to resources. The need for self-dependency had never been nurtured in her life before homelessness. Furthermore, the need to sustain herself with the necessary help was now being met by the NGO. So, there was no immediate requirement for her to be self-sufficient; thus, being content with her present status was enough for her to survive as long as this status quo was maintained.

This chapter illustrates a few life stories where each participant enumerated how they lost their momentum towards a potentially more fulfilling future as they could not garner hope (generally understood as a primary driving force in one's life journey). Ayesha, Karunai, and Shankar have been struggling against social suffering since childhood. While grappling with the issues related to their advanced age and geriatric ailments, homelessness, and SMI, they have been generally satisfied with their present way of life. With no one to take care of them as they age further, they expressed concern about attempting a more independent or empowered life within the scope of their limited resources. Simultaneously, Bijon and Sujaya, after facing and struggling with scores of challenges all their life and having no significant familial or social relations, found it challenging to re-search "hope" for a meaningful tomorrow. All their stories have been threaded with their contentment in their present way of life. It was partially because the "present" appeared comparatively more fulfilling than their "past." It might also be because they might have lost that zeal to move against the current amidst the myriads of suffering. The following chapter will enunciate further the role of "hope" as a way of life among these individuals who have suffered and survived homelessness and SMI towards recovery and empowerment.

5 Narratives of Recovery and Empowerment

In Chapter 3, we could observe that amidst intense social suffering owing to patriarchal power processes or geriatric issues, the participants generally indicated a lack of *hope* for a better future. Similarly, in Chapter 4, although the participants initially transcended the overwhelming impact of social suffering, their hope for a better future took a jolt due to growing age and the absence of a meaningful relational world with a significant other. Thus, in the last two chapters, we see that the relative lack of "hope" played a critical role in obtruding or slowing down their "upward mobilisation" towards recovery and empowerment. Therefore, this chapter examines how "hope" as a significant component may catalyse recovery and empowerment in HMI persons.

The following five life stories will explore how hope, as a way of life (with its source lying either in oneself or in significant others), remained core to the life journey of the participants towards recovery and empowerment despite social suffering or challenges to recovery and empowerment experienced by them. The stories of "Damayanti," "Chethana," "Pushpavalli," and "Pradeepto" would showcase how "hope embedded in the self" had become the driving factor in their process of recovery and empowerment. At the same time, "Snigdha's" story would situate the *source of hope in the relationship* with the significant other.

Damayanti

Damayanti was the first participant whom I interviewed on starting the fieldwork. The powerful features, stoic calm, and composed demeanour reflected the life of dignity that she had lived until very recently. She was lovingly addressed as Bhagavati by the counsellors and caregivers since that was the name she told them when she first came to the shelter house.

Monday to Friday, she used to drape a saree like the good old days while she went to teach at that school the NGO arranged for her. Had I seen her outside the shelter house, it would have been beyond my imagination that she underwent such life-changing storms.

When I approached her for the interview, she readily agreed to participate. The first question she asked me before I could tell her anything about my

DOI: 10.4324/9781032662053-5

research was, "what made this health condition happen?" I explained to her the biological and psychological causes that may lead to SMI. She inferred that psychological reasons had played a more significant role in her case. Throughout the interview, she maintained a calm expression. However, at specific points, while talking about her teaching experiences and her students, her face would light up, and her eyes would twinkle. At the end of an almost two-hour interview, she thanked me spontaneously for talking to her and listening to her patiently. She exclaimed with a sigh of relief, "I am feeling light after sharing all these years of pain with you."

Damayanti was the eldest sister of three brothers. Like any other suburban middle-class Bengali girl, she had a normal childhood. Her father worked at the railways while her mother was a house maker. Damayanti started teaching at a high school after graduating as an average but sincere student. Later she earned a degree in teachers' training as well and got married to a fellow teacher who taught in the primary section. They had a son together. Things were stable. However, during his teenage, her son started protesting his father's drinking and gambling behaviour which Damayanti chose to adjust to and compromise with for the family's sake. But when her son decided to move out of the house because it was affecting his studies, Damayanti supported him. The struggle of the single mother thus started, "I also left home with him. I just depended on my job. That is when the disaster of my life began. The more I tried to protect my son against it, the more I got affected."

Aspects of Social Suffering Associated with the Process of "Becoming" HMI Person Shaped by Familial and Socio-political Context

After separating from her husband, Damayanti ignored the societal frowns to support her son. She exclaimed, "The society never stopped judging and criticising. It even tried to take advantage of me, especially on financial matters, thinking me to be naïve and unprotected." She sent her son to the best colleges and universities. She played all possible roles as a mother. Damayanti supported him in all his life's decisions, including marriage, taking up jobs away from home, and settling abroad. However, when it was his turn to take care of his mother, Damayanti found herself all alone, like always.

> I lived in a rented house, so there were many questions from others. The neighbours tried intimidating me. I felt secure when he (my son) was around, but he left for college soon after his class XII. My landlord started rumouring about me that I did not clean up the place properly; I left it dirty. He used to create much fuss about my staying there alone. I was often asked why I lived alone! I am married, but I do not live with my husband. This was something frequently asked by neighbourhood women.

The contact with the son had already started fading down by this time. After teaching for 32 years, she retired a year after her son moved to the USA with his wife. Soon after, her mother passed away, who used to be a strong pillar of support for her. One of her brothers urged her to stay with them instead of living alone. But her experience of staying there with them made her feel like a burden to them. It kept adding to her already low mood due to cumulative losses (her son's shift to the USA, retirement, and her mother's death).

Damayanti was not able to recollect how or when her mental health started deteriorating. However, she identified an incident where she left home without any reason and was rendered lost. She recollected, "It all started suddenly. This happened once earlier. Yes, I left home and went to Katihar. Thankfully there were some good-hearted people there. They cared for me, treated me, and helped me return home."

To gain clarity on the signs of her mental health condition, in hindsight, Damayanti thought it was the accumulating stressors which precipitated the SMI. The signs went unnoticed and therefore undiagnosed and untreated, "I think I used to think a lot, to an extreme state, about me living alone, my son not being able to come there, retirement, my mother's death." After she left home for the first time, though her brother took her to a general physician, she was not provided with any medication. Thus, the symptoms persisted, and she again left home in an actively symptomatic phase. After being rescued from the streets by the NGO, her brother refused to take her back home and provide her shelter, treatment, or care. Damayanti felt the health condition had claimed a lot from her in all domains of her life.

> It hurts [her eyes well up]. Because of my health condition, I cannot mix up with people naturally. I want to, but I am not able to. I am very selective with whom I talk to, but it was not like this before the health condition. I have lost touch with anyone I ever knew. I could have been into a much healthier life, taking care of myself on my own [sighs]. A much smoother experience than the life I am living now. Some way or the other, I would have survived at my brother's place. Life would not have been this uncertain, especially the financial condition. I have suffered a lot and am still suffering from that (mental health condition).

While her first episode of SMI went unidentified and untreated, the relapse brought her out of the home. This time she ended up on the streets of Kolkata, roaming around for days. Finally, she was rescued from the streets of Kolkata by the local police in a disoriented, dishevelled condition.

> This time I left home, and it was all blank from there. I do not remember. I was just roaming around like a beggar on the streets. I do not know how I reached this far because I do not know if I had any money. And while I was roaming the streets, the police took me and brought me here. But I do not remember that also. After I was brought here, I could remember things from my past.

Following a few months of treatment, she could gradually reveal her name, address, etc. However, as mentioned earlier, on taking her back to her brother's, he refused to take any further responsibility for her. On top of this, she had also lost all her relevant documents, bank papers, etc., while she was on the streets (she had them on her. Iswar Sankalpa, however, took the initiative to retrieve the documents that helped her access her pension once again). However, she could not recollect the suffering she experienced while on the streets. But the fact that she became homeless because of a mental health condition and was not forced out of her home by relatives kept her confidence alive in her family. She still hoped her son could not take her to the USA; it was against the custom there.

> I would like to live with my son, but I have heard that it is not a practice in America to live with your parents, maybe because of that, he would not take me there with him [she tried to force a smile].

As a mother, she proved how much she could sacrifice to provide her son a comfortable life by ignoring her socio-culturally rooted mothering instincts. Despite all attempts, her son could not be contacted until very recently (in November 2017, three years after being rescued). However, he refused to take responsibility despite being back in India.

Deep inside, she knew that her dream of staying with her son during her last days was far from materialised. She thus simultaneously hoped for a home where she could live independently and self-sufficiently. For her having a roof above her head did not mean home. She still considered herself homeless. Homelessness for Damayanti was

> a very negative feeling, a bitter one; there is a constant emptiness within you (khali lage mon ta, shunyo). While my colleagues have four-storeyed houses, I have become homeless in a shelter house. I feel helpless.

Challenges to the Process of Recovery and Empowerment

Damayanti's helplessness was magnified when challenges manifested in various forms on her way to recovery and empowerment. Though clinically recovered, she could not take the risk of moving forward towards an independent life. She wanted to, but her age became a constraint, "I am not that young now that I would be able to take care of all my needs and requirements on my own." Furthermore, the loss of her financial documents further stopped her from accessing her pension account. She exclaimed, "Some of the money has been recovered and transferred. They are trying to retrieve the pension account and fixed deposit account. But I am not hoping much."

Despite acknowledging every bit of help received from the NGO, she accepted that it was quite challenging to stay among those who were yet to recover, "It is quite challenging to live with these girls here. For example, we share toilets, and many of them are very poor in hygiene; it is tricky to cope with these things." Moreover, she had been one of those individuals who had made decisions for herself all her life. She, thus, found it difficult when she had to follow the mandate of the NGO.

> I can tell you about some small things. For example, say if I feel like having a cup of Horlicks, I cannot have it here because I cannot drink alone in front of so many other girls. It is mostly because of our situation here; the rules and regulations would not allow me to have it.

Process of Recovery and Empowerment

Damayanti expressed her gratitude for being rescued from the streets by the police. She felt obliged that Iswar Sankalpa accepted her unconditionally, providing her with a space to stay, and making all the essential resources accessible, which her own blood relations refused.

> I was just roaming around like a beggar on the streets. I do not know how I reached this far because I do not know if I had any money. And while I was roaming the streets, the police took me and brought me here. Taking medicines, the help and cooperation from this NGO and the care they have provided me helped me to do this.

Throughout the interview, Damayanti talked about how she was perturbed about losing all her documents and that it made her financial condition unstable. She, nevertheless, acknowledged the immense role the NGO had been playing in trying to retrieve the documents so that she could access her pension account once again.

Damayanti identified the help she got from the NGO in getting a part-time teaching job at a local school.

> Ms K (a social worker) helped me to get this job. She talked to the headmaster, explained my situation, and vouched for me. She gave me confidence, motivated me a lot, brought me books before school, and took me to the school before joining to introduce me to all the other staff. They have been very accommodating.

Further, she acknowledged the support and respect she had been getting from her colleagues ever since she joined. It reassured and validated her self-esteem and proficiency as a teacher, which she feared had succumbed to her health condition. Finally, Damayanti expressed her contentment with regaining her physical and cognitive abilities that had once been compromised because of the untreated SMI, followed by her days on the streets. She recollected, "I was not able to do anything previously, but with the medication now, I can function like before."

At present, she felt satisfied to some extent with the chances of the pension being retrieved. However, she knew with her lifelong struggle that financial independence would be essential for her to thrive the days outside the NGO.

> Whatever has been recovered is enough for me to survive. It is hard earned money. So, it would be good if I get them back. Moreover, it would help me to live independently, to rent a house and get a house help to stay with me.

The experience of going back to teaching once again boosted that dormant self-esteem.

> I am enjoying teaching like before; it is very peaceful. I am teaching class V now. The school headmaster asked me to teach that class because they are coming from the primary section; they need a solid base in science, so I am teaching them only.

Damayanti singled out that living among the symptomatic co-residents was the most challenging adjustment she made while living at the shelter house; she, nevertheless, identified the positive side of living at the NGO, especially at her age.

> There are also some positive sides to living here because so many of them are around. For example, whenever I feel unwell, I have someone or the other to take care of me, which would not be possible if I lived alone.

As a teacher, regaining her identity helped her feel socially relevant and resourceful.

> The students are very friendly, and they are quite restless and young. They will not ask for your permission. They would take chalk and go to the blackboard to solve a sum even before I could request them. I am like a grandma to them [her face lights up with a bright smile].

She narrated the experience of an old student tracking her and visiting her at the NGO. She was overwhelmed, but it helped her validate her self-esteem.

> A student of mine came to visit me here after she learned about my condition. She came with her husband, and she brought food and a

saree with her. When I was tracking those lost documents, she came to know about me somehow. She was unsure if I was there and contacted different old age homes to find me. Then she found me here. I impacted her life and made her search for me [smiles as tears roll down her eyes].

And it kept the hope alive in her that as a teacher, she would always be a resource to society, contributing to the lives of her students. It gave purpose and meaning to her existence, even amidst experiencing the marginalisation of extreme forms, "I think I still have an impact on the children I am teaching now. As long as I would teach, I would affect my students."

Struggling all her life against the patriarchal powers of Indian society, Damayanti did not have much to hope for at the dusk of her life.

I think I myself, am the source of my strength. I hope to stay healthy till my last breath and be self-sufficient, not depending on others. I cannot afford to depend on others; that is all I want. My mother cooked her last meal, had a stroke in the evening and died. I want my death to be like that! Silent and peaceful. I don't want to disturb others much [sighs].

After being betrayed by all the familial relations, she found strength in herself to spend these last days as contently as possible at this juncture. She had spent most of her adulthood being financially empowered. She thus knew the importance of living a self-sufficient, independent life. All she hoped for now was to stay physically and mentally healthy. After being dejected by blood relations in all possible manner, she just looked forward to a peaceful death without becoming a "problem" to anyone anymore.

Chethana

Chethana was a 39-year-old unmarried woman from a lower SES, rural family in Andhra Pradesh. She was the youngest of three sisters and one brother. After failing to pass her 10th exams, Chethana took training in tailoring for one year and mastered embroidery skills. Then, she started working as a sweeper in the village primary school, using her tailoring skills on the sides. However, life changed for Chethana following her father's death when she got affected by a serious mental illness.

Chethana has been a resident of The Banyan since 2008. Amidst her hectic schedule, it was tricky for her to get one or two hours to sit with me and talk. We exchanged pleasantries now and then since she was proficient in Hindi. I learned much about her life in those few minutes of "chats." Nevertheless, she did manage to find time for me and tell me her story in detail on a Sunday afternoon, the day she did not need to go to her work.

Aspects of Social Suffering Associated with the Process of "Becoming"
HMI Person Shaped by Familial and Socio-political Context

Life had been kind to Chethana for as long as she could remember. Following school, when she started earning money, it gave her a new outlook on her self-worth. It made her feel important when she could contribute to her family financially. However, a few years later, when her father passed away due to cancer, Chethana became extremely upset, with frequent weeping spells.

> I was taken to the government hospital and given medicine and an electric shock. Then I was discharged from the hospital. Then one day, I was to visit one of my sisters. I had to take a train, but I do not know how I forgot everything and where to go. I boarded the wrong train. I ended up in Chennai. I was roaming the streets. I do not remember what I was eating or where I was staying. Finally, someone brought me here to The Banyan. That was in 2003.

She was rescued from the streets in a dishevelled state by The Banyan and treated there for two months. Once she started responding to the medicines, she could recollect her address. She was sent back home. However, back home, she was rejected by her brother and sister-in-law. She still remembered them saying, "why have you come back here! Go back to where you were staying!." Nevertheless, her mother stood by her, and both of them struggled to make ends meet.

Chethana tried to get her previous job back at the school. However, she was no longer allowed there because of her mental health diagnosis. The continuous rejection and labelling humiliated her and made her feel dehumanised and dejected. She continued experiencing the brunt of mental health conditions in all domains of life beyond its symptoms.

> When I went to find work, they were like, "how would you work! You are a pagal (mad person)! You have a mental problem; we cannot give you work!." They taunted me, saying, "you are too fat to work, your mood changes, you are not good for any work" [tears rolled down, and we stopped the interview until she could gather herself back].

In the neighbourhood also, the non-acceptance was extremely evident. She recalled, "I used to go to the market, and people would point at me saying, 'this girl is pagal (mad), she is mental.' Some neighbours would not allow me to enter their house!"

Her mother worked as a labourer at a construction site. Chethana joined her. In between, she was provided with her medicines consistently by the NGO through postal order and a little monetary allowance of 100 rupees every three months. But her sister-in-law did not make it any easier for her to stay home.

I used to fetch drinking water from the tube well outside the home. But my sister-in-law would throw away that water. She would not let anyone use the water that I fetched. I had no infection on my hands, right? So, why not drink that water? But she would not understand! She made my utensils separate, and that made me feel horrible. Finally, my brother gave my mother and me a room to stay in. My brother gave us the ration but separated our kitchen. We managed somehow.

However, the status quo did not last long for them. Both the mother and daughter fell ill with jaundice at the same time. Both lost their job. And her mother could not survive the late diagnosis, and due to lack of proper treatment and adequate care, she passed away in 2008. After her mother's death, her brother and sister-in-law refused her shelter at her own house.

One of my sisters took me along with her, as my sister-in-law did not allow me to stay there. But there used to be fights at her home with her husband regarding my stay with them. Her husband was against me staying there.

By now, Chethana had had enough of the humiliation. She felt betrayed by all her siblings. Even the community was not tolerant of her diagnosis. And thus, she chose to take charge of her own life.

One day I called The Banyan and told them that my mother was dead and that I had nowhere else to go. So they asked me to come back here. My sister brought me here after that. Since then, I have been staying here.

While the first time Chethana became homeless was during the symptomatic phase. This time, the circumstances ultimately forced her to choose a shelter house over staying with her relatives. The extreme form of humiliation and alienation that she experienced from her relatives and the patriarchal society drove her to the shelter house. Even when she tried to have an independent living, because she was a woman, she also experienced a threat in that attempt.

There was a neighbour, he was almost 45 years old. He was married. He would come to me and tell me, "come to me, I will have you. You are pagal (mad), and no one would marry you. Why don't you come to me!." I got terrified. I don't dare stay alone after that. I just want to be safe. I am safe here.

With her share of negative experiences in the community as a woman, Chethana chose to stay at the shelter house and came to terms with her meaning of home. She conceived the shared house as home because that was where she felt safe and understood.

Process of Recovery and Empowerment

Since 2008 Chethana has been working as a tailor in the vocational training centre of the NGO. For the last year, she was recruited at a private hospital where she works as a health care worker.

At present, Chethana has been living in a shared house with three other residents under the supervision of a healthcare worker. She experienced immense satisfaction with her current status as an empowered individual with an improved quality of life at the shared house. Unlike the women's shelter house, where she had to reside with symptomatic co-residents, she found the shared house a more peaceful abode. As mentioned earlier, she conceptualised it as equivalent to home because she enjoyed her independence and strong mutual bond with her co-residents.

> I am satisfied here. I live in a shared home now and like it there [smiles]. It has more privacy than the shelter house. I have my bed; we watch tv, go to movies, and go shopping; I have freedom, and I feel happy. If I go out and live alone, I will have to cook and do all the chores. Here I can share my work with others. I can balance household chores and work with their help. Alone it would be challenging. Since we all share the work, it is easier to stay there.

Like most other rehabilitated individuals, Chethana felt obliged to the NGO for providing her with the safety and security that her family had refused her. Thus, instead of trying to find meaningful relationships with her family of origin, Chethana accepted the NGO, its residents, and the service providers as her family. They supported her unconditionally when she needed it the most.

> Whatever I have is The Banyan. Rather than trying to find a life outside, I would stay with this family and try to do something better for those suffering. I do not need my siblings [eyes well up].

Her co-residents had become her new family with whom she once again deciphered meaning to her existence. She felt relevant and resourceful among them, and the feelings were mutual.

> Everyone there speaks Telegu. We chat, come to work and return in the evening. I like staying with people. I do not want to stay alone. There is one who does not work at all. We scold her. I feel closest to Mariyam. She guides and helps me if I do not know something [laughs heartily].

Years of fighting the society and system had left Chethana with deeply embedded insights. She knew that no one would if she did not fight for herself. Her composure and persistence had been her weapon in all her struggles, "I get the strength to keep on fighting from myself. I tell myself to keep patience. Problems would get over eventually."

Chethana was aware of the need to remain financially empowered to secure a stable, self-dependent future. She knew that if she lost her "employability," she would probably be again dispensable. However, she did not want to risk it, "I would continue my medication. I would go to work, earn money. I pray to God that let me be in this state so that I can stay healthy and work. I want to settle down eventually."

Life had made Chethana aware of her limitations. She had learnt the hard way how to overcome her vulnerabilities.

> People think that since I am mentally ill, I cannot work even when I am well. I work as a healthcare worker. But I am still addressed as a client. I want to get past this point and be acknowledged only as a healthcare worker.

While she is aware of her responsibilities, society is not. It still recognised her only as an individual with a mental health condition. She wanted to establish her identity beyond that, and she hoped for a future where she would be acknowledged for her work, not the health condition she survived.

Pushpavalli

Pushpavalli grew up with his two younger brothers having an ordinary childhood like most others. The suffering that life offered her was well within her tolerance threshold until she got diagnosed with a mental health condition. This was followed by the death of her husband within a year of her marriage. After this, she was forced to give away her newborn daughter for adoption. For the last seven years, Pushpavalli had been staying with The Banyan and trying to gather the pieces of her life together towards a meaningful future.

Aspects of Social Suffering Associated with the Process of "Becoming" HMI Person Shaped by Familial and Socio-political Context

Pushpavalli remembered her father being a drunkard, but it was a typical affair in their neighbourhood. However, there were days when he would come home drunk and beat her mother. Pushpavalli would fight with him on such occasions to save her mother. He died when she was 14. Pushpavalli had to leave school, being the eldest of three siblings, to afford the family. She studied till the eighth standard. Life was challenging because of the financial dearth but inconsequential until she got affected by SMI. It went undiagnosed and untreated, and during a symptomatic episode, she came out of home, wandered, and ended up in Chennai. Rescued by The Banyan, after treatment, she could be reinstated back home.

> When I was twenty, I suddenly had those symptoms: I came out of the house, wandered on the streets, and ended up in Chennai to see the actor. I stayed at The Banyan for one year. After getting the treatment, I could remember my address and family. I went back home. I was distraught having this diagnosis. No one had any idea what this health condition was. There were a lot of financial burdens accompanied by this.

Though she went back home, the recurring cost that the treatment of a life-long diagnosis of a mental health condition was too much for them to bear. So, no sooner than later, the treatment got discontinued. But, with no relapse, she continued with the job that she had been doing previously.

A few years later, Pushpavalli got married. It, she recollected, was the happiest moment of her life. She enjoyed a cordial loving relationship with her in-laws. But that did not last more than a year. Her husband committed suicide over a familial discord just after a year of marriage.

> He (his husband) committed suicide. He took money against my jewellery for his business. My relatives got very angry with him. My mother's brother questioned him. My husband had wanted me to keep it confidential, but I casually mentioned it to my mother. I never thought things would become this ugly. My uncle accused him of not being able to take care of me. He said my husband had no rights on my jewellery as they were given to me. In our culture, taking money against jewellery is not something ordinary. My husband was a sensitive man. He could not tolerate all those acquisitions. He felt insulted and committed suicide [by this time, she had started sobbing, unable to control her tears. She excused herself for a while and returned after a few minutes, gathering herself again].

Both Pushpavalli and her husband became victims of the ageless patriarchal practices. She considered herself responsible for his death. Being continuously blamed for his death by his relatives did not ease the feeling of guilt or grief. Her in-laws did not allow her back home. Eight months pregnant then, Pushpavalli had a relapse. She gave premature birth to a baby girl. While no treatment was sought for her relapse, her family, on the other side, decided on her behalf that the newborn would be better off if given up for adoption.

> I gave my child away for adoption. I delivered the child at home, but I was unable to take care of the child. My mother and my aunt decided to give her away for adoption. They persuaded me, telling me that I would not be able to take care of my child. I agreed. I thought she should not suffer like me. She should get a proper education and a good life.

Pushpavalli was persuaded that she would not be an ideal caregiver for her daughter. When her daughter was given away for adoption, her mother sent her back to The Banyan since she did not have money to treat the ailing daughter. In retrospect, Pushpavalli had been repenting her decision for all these years. She lamented the loss of her child and felt dejected about being denied the experience of mothering her child.

> It was the wrong decision. I should not have given up my child for adoption. Now that I am doing better with medication, I repent my decision. If I had asserted my mother's decision, I could have had her. I should not have abandoned her [she could not meet my eyes as she talked about how she lamented her decision].

Left with the feeling of being betrayed by her familial relations for denying her shelter and care, Pushpavalli had come to terms with considering the shelter house as her home. Now that she had been living in a shared house as part of the "Home Again" project, she had been able to re-establish her meaning of the home that had been robbed from her earlier. With two kids staying with them at that house, Pushpavalli had been putting out some of her unquenched thirst for motherhood.

> I have a home. I live in a shared house that feels like home. Home means family, love, and sharing. Two kids are staying with us in the shared household. Their mothers live in Kovalam. It feels good to have those kids with us. It feels like we are sharing our love, a bond. I feed them, play with them, and tell them not to do certain things. Then, in the evening, they wait for me to come back, and we have dinner together and watch tv. All these are making that place a home for me.

Challenges to the Process of Recovery and Empowerment

In the past seven years that she had been with The Banyan, Pushpavalli tried to go out of the safe perimeters of the NGO and live independently with the help of the job opportunities they sought. But, every time, Pushpavalli experienced poor adherence to the treatment regime. On both occasions in which she had lived without the supervision of a caregiver, Pushpavalli had stopped her medication when she felt she had been doing fine. And thus, she was, to a certain extent, sceptical of living alone without anyone with her.

> Every time I go back, I stop my medication. And whenever I stop my medicines, I again become ill. I was told not to stop the medicines. But I thought I could stop taking the medication since I was doing well. This (stopping the medicine) has happened twice.

Furthermore, considering the vulnerabilities a woman holds based on her gender norms, it was a concern for Pushpavalli to stay beyond these secure boundaries.

> There is no safety when you are staying alone. Men try to take advantage of you when you are alone. For a woman, security becomes an issue if one is staying alone. If you have to stay alone, then you need to have some good friends around you.

And so, in her mind, Pushpavalli had etched a plan to wait for a few more years and then go out of the NGO setting with some of her friends from here, rent a place and stay together on their own.

Process of Recovery and Empowerment

Pushpavalli felt that The Banyan had been her proxy family for all these years and had done everything her family should have done for her. It had given her access to the right resources and had rebuilt her trust in herself to become self-sufficient.

> They helped me a lot. What my family had to do for me, The Banyan did for me. They have trained me to live a life by not depending on anyone. I work in the canteen. I make tea and coffee, and I serve them. I cook also.

And this newly developed trust in self helped her to look forward to a future where she considered herself living independently, fully aware of the challenges that it would mean, "I would like to go out and live independently. For me, independence is meeting my own needs and living the life based on my personal choice." With her prior experiences working in various settings, Pushpavalli was confident about finding a job when she moved out of the NGO. She wanted a better-paid job to help her meet all those wishes that had remained unfulfilled because of the lifelong struggle with money.

> I would have to make arrangements for my food, clothes and shelter. I would also like to buy some pieces of jewellery. Unfortunately, I don't earn much now to meet all my wishes. When I go out, I will search for a job which would pay me better.

After all these years of suffering, Pushpavalli wanted nothing but the essentials of her life – some happiness that life had always denied her and a steady income. However, she wondered whether she would ever find that coveted happiness since her happiness had sublimed with sacrificing her right to motherhood!

Pradeepto

Orphaned in childhood, Pradeepto was brought up primarily by his elder brother and uncle. His brother took care of all his financial requirements. He stayed with his uncle's family since his brother had a transferable job. While he was in the fifth standard, Pradeepto suffered from meningitis. As a result, he had to discontinue his schooling. Early in life, he started earning his pocket money by delivering milk packets in the neighbourhood. A few years later, when Pradeepto was in his early twenties, he found a better-paying job. After that, things were stable until he fell into the practice of abusing alcohol, and life took the worst possible turn he could expect.

Aspects of Social Suffering Associated with the Process of "Becoming"
HMI Person Shaped by Familial and Socio-political Context

Pradeepto was introduced to alcohol by his cousins. However, he began abusing it and became an addict. With no one to stop, take care of and supervise him, the addiction eventually took over his self-control, and he also lost his job.

> I started consuming alcohol. One of my cousins used to drink at home. He used to force me to drink with him, but I tried to avoid it. But later, when I started working, I fell into the habit of drinking. It increased more after I left my job. There was a time when I would stop whatever I was doing and open the bottle as soon as it was 12 p.m. at the clock. Whatever I was earning was spent on alcohol [sighs!].

When his brother knew about this, he became concerned and asked him to shift to Patna, where he was posted. Although Pradeepto did that, he fell seriously ill there. So he decided to move back to Kolkata and join the job he left. But there were no vacancies at that moment. And the lack of employment and appropriate supervision from caregivers thus once again reopened the vicious loop of alcohol abuse. At this time, his cousins started having tiffs with him over property issues.

> After I came back to Kolkata, my cousins started abusing me physically. They wanted me to leave the house. They would beat me every night. I filed cases against them at the police station, but the police took no steps.

Helpless by the apathy of the stakeholders at the systemic level and under the influence of alcohol, Pradeepto did not get in touch with his brother and started living on the streets, and thus began his life of homelessness. (While it was unclear from his narrative whether Pradeepto was already suffering the symptoms of mental health condition before he left home. However, it may be safe to assume under the given circumstances, he might have been struggling with low mood, which, coupled with alcohol abuse, led to further deterioration of his mental health.)

> I came out of the house and started living in front of a tea stall. I stayed on the streets for almost three years. My condition deteriorated because of my drinking. I used to abuse everyone when I was drunk.

Though his cousin's wife provided him with some money daily, instead of buying food with that, he used to purchase alcohol. And life on the street was not any kinder to him, "There was no place to sleep. There were a tea stall and a food stall, and they would give me food. Life was painful. I have tolerated rain and sun for three years out there." Since he was almost provoked to leave home and choose homelessness, for Pradeepto, the meaning of home was no more related to his family, nor could he consider the shelter-house as home. Nevertheless, he was ready to reclaim what was home to him.

> This (the NGO) has sheltered me, but this is not home. I have a home, but I have been forcefully removed from there. I want to complain about my cousins again, and I want to go back to my house.

Process of Recovery and Empowerment

Identified at a medical camp organised by Iswar Sankalpa along with the Kolkata Municipality Corporation, Pradeepto was rescued for staying at the male shelter house "Marudyan." He was primarily considered for in-house treatment and rehabilitation to deal with his chronic alcohol abuse. At the outreach programme, chances of relapse for substance abuse individuals were much higher as the caregivers had identified at the NGO from past experiences. Though he was sceptical at first, gradually, he settled down. He acknowledged the help received from the NGO, "When they brought me here, I did not want to come. I did not know what place this would be, where they were taking me. But now that I am here, I know what they do."

While Pradeepto received resources from the NGO, simultaneously, at the same time, he started taking action to come back into the mainstream. He started with little but very significant steps, "After coming here, when I started feeling better with medicines, I started waking up early and doing exercises." Pradeepto had insights into his potential, and thus when the NGO found him a job, he pushed for something better.

> Initially, they found me a job at a roadside eatery. But they (the employer) would not give me money but food twice. So what's the point of working there? Then I told Didi (meaning sister, the shelter coordinator) that I wanted to visit my previous employer for a job. I knew they would help me. So I went there with her.

And his instincts turned out to be right. He was re-employed by his previous employer, and at present, he is employed as a personal assistant. Content with the respectable status of his job and his relationship with his employer, Pradeepto had now been thinking about what next.

> Now, I must have an Aadhar card, as that's mandatory. Then I would reclaim my share in the property. I need to discuss with my brother how I should proceed. He had come here to see me here.

With his brother's help, he planned to access his right to his property, but for that, he wanted to wait for some more time. In between, he tried to continue his current job and nurture his newfound dependable relationships. While he felt his friends from his past had failed him when he needed them the most, that feeling of being betrayed did not stop him from rebuilding a social network.

While Pradeepto was aware of all he had lost to his mental health condition and the betrayal of his family members, it had not let him lose self-belief even in the face of extreme crisis.

> I have my inner strength, which has helped me to fight against all those odds. I would keep on doing that. I had a mental health condition, so I had to take medicine. I took the initiative to return to the mainstream when I became well.

And that remained his source of strength in his journey back to the mainstream.

Snigdha

Snigdha was one of those few residents at the shelter house who had been rescued from the streets while conducting my fieldwork there. High on irritability, she was resistant and uncooperative when I first met her. Sitting on a wooden bench at one corner of the corridor, for hours, she would mutter to herself about her fate, the apathy the entire world had shown towards her and being "locked out" from the rest of the world against her will "with some mad people."

Snigdha, 36 years old, had just recovered from malaria and was still having active symptoms of SMI. She used to be very weak and hungry most of the time. Occasionally, she would demand tea which she was refused as they followed a fixed schedule for all the residents. To retaliate, she would refuse to participate in any shelter activities. This had almost become a cycle for nearly a month. Every day, I used to sit with her for some time to listen to her complaints against the rest of the world – her parents, her husband, and the shelter house caretaker. I asked no questions, but just listened to her talking. The only thing I could do for her was to arrange with a caregiver to give her some in-between food meals. The reason stated was that she was recovering from her physical ailment. But I wanted to use it as a positive reinforcer to engage her in socialisation.

Soon, she started participating in some regular chores, actively taking responsibility, and performing in the functional-literacy classes. Before long, Snigdha was learning steps for a dance performance they would present to some visiting donors. Not only did she learn, rehearse sincerely, and perform it, she told me in one of our daily pep talks, "I want to learn this because when I would go out, I would be able to teach this at least to one child."

I interviewed her during the first week of November, exactly two months after my first interaction with her. The distinctively visible changes in her were speaking volumes of her resilience, that no matter what, she would fight against the current, swimming towards the mainstream.

Aspects of Social Suffering Associated with the Process of "Becoming" HMI Person Shaped by Familial and Socio-political Context

Eldest of seven siblings, all sisters, Snigdha had been a witness and victim of domestic violence ever since she was a little girl. A physically abusive father not only tortured the mother and her daughters for not bearing him a son but gradually drove her to leave her family and her children behind. Left to take care of her younger sisters, Snigdha, very early in her life, became the prey of her male relatives. Snigdha stood face to face with the harsh realities of life and thus started her fight against it. Falling in love at the naïve age of 16, she started dreaming of that life of love and peace that she could never have at her father's place. She trusted her admirer enough to leave the house with him to start a family. But, regarding caste issues, he refused to marry her.

> My partner and I never had a legal marriage. There were caste issues. He (her partner) was from Bihar; they are of businessman caste, and we were Brahmin. He took me to the temple and put sindhur (vermillion) on my hair [a Hindu ritual performed during wedding ceremonies].

Though they lived under the same roof for 15 years, they never got married legally. After having one son and one daughter with him, she was forced to abort when she became pregnant for the third time and the following three times. Though it was her child, her words held no value to them.

> After the birth of my first two children, they made me abort. In the fourth month of pregnancy, my mother-in-law and my husband would make me abort the child because I did not agree to do the ligation. They abused me and used to curse me.

She always wanted to have many children, believing that the child would bring happiness and peace to her family.

I used to think children bring happiness to families, and I thought my children would bring peace and joy to my family. But, unfortunately, there has never been happiness or peace in my life from childhood until now. Instead, there are jealousy and dissension everywhere.

Trying to balance her life amongst her children and the lingering financial crisis, she broke down gradually, facing the everyday physical abuse from her husband.

Every day we fought. He had bought a shack at a slum, apparently for me to stay with the children. But when you have a home, you expect some peace in there. There was no peace. Even the basic amenities were not there, not even a bathroom.

Years of dehumanisation and subjugation forced Snigdha to leave her household and her children behind one day after being severely battered. Disenchanted with the concept of family and home, Snigdha chose the streets over the abusive house, "Home is somewhere where you are responsible for each other, living with the loved ones, a place where the company gives you happiness."

She had to take up prostitution as a livelihood since Snigdha was not left with any option, and she left it when she realised she was pregnant.

I had no place to go. I got no shelter, I tried, but nobody would give me a place to sleep and live for free. So, I went to this "line neighbourhood." You get to book a room for yourself and your customer based on per hour. So, I used to book for 24 hours and have as many customers as possible. This line (prostitution) was the only way to save my life: to have food and shelter at night. But then I became pregnant. However, I decided to keep the child at any cost. So, I left that line once I became pregnant.

Her intense love for her unborn child did not let her abort the child even when she was not aware of the identity of the father. Instead, she chose to fight society to protect it.

Society would not have minded having the child from a thief, so why not my child? I thought somehow or the other, I would raise her, she would be walking with me on this journey, and maybe someday she would find her relatives; perhaps her beauty, her youth would make someone fall in love with her.

Snigdha started rag-picking when she left her previous job. Then, at the advanced stage of her pregnancy, she had no option but to beg. She delivered the child on the streets and reared up the child against all the odds.

After she was born, I did not go for rag-picking even. I started to sell lozenges. If you buy lozenges for 100rs, you can earn 200 rupees by selling them. I sold them during the day and then freshened up and sat with the child in front of a temple or mosque and begged. Sometimes you would have to fight with the other pavement dwellers to survive.

But Snigdha lost all her strength and courage to fight any longer when that child was taken away from her by the child-welfare committee.

I initially thought it would do good for her. If she had to live on the streets, she would have to undergo the same sufferings I would suffer through, arranging all the basic needs, from food to shelter. She would have to do it all as I had done since childhood. But if she lived in the NGO home, she might live a better life than on the streets. But they do not let me meet my child. If you lose something that belongs to you, it hurts.

The immense feeling of being betrayed by the familial relations followed by the society and system left her emotionally exhausted. When she was denied the experience of mothering her child, her last resort, it was the final straw. She held the incident of her child being taken away as the factor that precipitated the deterioration of her mental health.

It happened after they took away the child. But I do not remember much of it. I guess I stopped eating, sleeping or taking care of myself. I always was angry. First, they sent me home, but I tried to set everything on fire. Then they brought me here.

After the child had been sent to a care home, Snigdha was rescued from the streets and returned to her family (of procreation). However, the family brought her to the NGO and refused to take on her responsibility.

Challenges to the Process of Recovery and Empowerment

Behind the closed gates of the shelter-house, Snigdha considered herself caged. She was stuck there because they were not allowing her to go outside. Locked up against her will was making her even more helpless and restless. She felt humiliated because she found herself unheard within the hierarchical structure of the NGO.

I participate in the activities here because it makes time pass. If I sit idly, I ponder what I would do with my life, my child, and my future. Those thoughts keep coming back, and I get worried and upset since I do not have answers. So, I keep myself busy. But this is not my life. I do not like it here. Not at all. I am here because I have no way out. The moment they would let me go, I would leave.

Process of Recovery and Empowerment

While Snigdha had no social support outside the NGO and disliked staying at the shelter house, she found the company of her co-residents, who had re-established themselves back into the mainstream, immensely inspiring. Their success made her hopeful about a future outside the shelter house.

> I genuinely respect these women who have started their lives here from scratch and now, living independently, have made a bank balance of ten thousand rupees. They are great. They had no identity, no address, yet, they have done this. Their success gives me hope, and their stories inspire me. Imagine doing this when you have no loved one beside you, stuck in a shelter house. But they have done it!

She mentioned that she participated in shelter activities to keep herself busy from worrying. Snigdha also considered those as learning opportunities for new skills, the skills she did not have a chance to learn earlier. She thought she might be able to use them for the betterment of her own life as well as the lives of others.

> Whatever I am learning here, at some point or other in my life, I would try to help another person to realise that. I might be able to earn something from that. That is why I engage myself with whatever they ask me to do.

Snigdha understood with clarity the need for her to become self-sufficient and self-dependent. However, she was not ready to return to her family until they received her with her due respect.

> If he can give me the respect I deserve from him, only then can I think of living there. Just think for once, I have undergone. They are now making fun of my situation, waiting to see what I would do with the child.

Though she missed her children, she also knew how they considered her a bad mother because that was what their father had taught them about her. And thus, she was not to appear weak in front of them. Even if she were allowed outside the shelter house to earn her livelihood, she would not provide them with money. Snigdha still suffered the feeling of betrayal that she experienced when her children did not stand up for her while their father abused her.

He (my husband) had indulged them, my children, to believe I am a terrible mother. They are doing well and growing up fine. However, never did they acknowledge my contribution in their life. I had earned more money, saved more from 2005 to 2014 and afforded them everything I could. I worked as an attendant at the centres. I did night duties. I had also been a hawker, which I have been later while living on the streets. But now? Now, I am the bad one!

With whatever little she was earning from her daily chores at the shelter house, Snigdha had gathered back her confidence that it would be enough for her to start life outside. But all she needed for that was the NGO's support. Her experience of staying self-sufficient in the harshest situations was her capital in planning any empowerment endeavour.

I am earning some money here. After some time, I would use that to start some business. I can be a hawker or something of that sort. I know how to make money. I would do business as I did before. I want to go out from this place for 12 hours in the day, do some work, earn money, and come back here at night for the shelter.

Snigdha needed to ensure for herself and her infant daughter a financially secure future where neither of them would be considered dispensable by society or family. For that, she was ready to take as much risk as required to establish a self-dependent identity.

At present, two years after being brought to the shelter house, Snigdha works at the bakery, a self-help group of the residents. She visited her daughter at the child-welfare home once every month and stayed in touch with her husband, in-laws, and children. But, parallelly, she had been looking forward to the day when she could independently sustain herself and her daughter outside the shelter house.

In this chapter, I have reconstructed the life story of a few of those participants who, in their struggle as HMI individuals, could gather "hope" as their "way of life" to move away from the margins back into mainstream society (or community life). Social suffering has been prevalent in all the stories collected during my fieldwork. A few got stuck at the barriers social suffering set on their pathways (Chapter 3). In contrast, others overcame those hurdles but lost the momentum to continue the struggle with the same intensity across the journey (Chapter 4). As we could note in these two previous chapters, besides social suffering owing to patriarchal power processes or other forms of relational hierarchies, the life-long challenges, the dual burden of homelessness and SMI, ageing, absence of significant social ties with others turned out to be some crucial aspects of their lives that made their future appear meaningless or less meaningful. However, the life story illustrated in this chapter explored how walking that extra mile "with hope" carried them further towards recovery and empowerment. The life story of

Damayanti, Chethana, Pushpavalli, and Pradeepto exemplified that the "hope embedded in the self" might be the catalyser in maintaining the momentum of the journey towards recovery and empowerment. At the same time, Snigdha's story reverberates how hope embedded in her relationship with her significant other (her infant child) became her source of strength.

In the following chapter, I will explore the significant role played by the service providers in initiating and maintaining the recovery and empowerment processes. In doing so, I would attempt to understand the processes that motivate the service providers to engage with a marginalised population like the HMI persons and the challenges the service providers need to overcome.

6 Experience of Service Providers

Factors of Motivation and Challenges

dātavyam iti yad dānaṁ dīyate nupakāriṇe
deśhe kāle cha pātre cha tad dānaṁ sāttvikaṁ smṛitam
(Serving unconditionally to the one who needs and deserves it, at the right
place and time, with the feeling that it is 'one's duty, is considered the nature
of goodness). Bhagavad Gita, 17/20

Mental health is unquestionably one of the many neglected issues in developing nations. Patel and Thara (2003) determined that the NGO sector bears a substantial amount of responsibility for bridging this gap. India has taken various initiatives on paper (signing the UNCRPD in 2006 and passing the Mental Healthcare Act of 2017) to meet the challenges posed by the growing number of untreated mentally ill citizens. But this gap is too wide to be filled so. Thus, the role of NGOs remains as relevant as it was 20 years ago. Although Patel and Thara (2003) emphasised their significance, they also emphasised the paucity of NGOs committed to serving the mentally ill population. However, the dedication of those working tirelessly in this field despite all obstacles (including a lack of funding) is never fully recognised.

It can be challenging to work in the field of mental illness, but it is even more difficult to assist those with mental illness who are also homeless. To begin with, the homeless population is extremely transient. In India, only the NGO sector has been involved in the community mental health rehabilitation of HMI individuals. Moreover, although diagnosing mental illness is not difficult, it remains critical. Additionally, a medical practitioner must be involved. Unfortunately, the ratio of psychiatrists to patients in India is grossly inadequate, making it difficult to find trained professionals for the NGO sector. In addition, the absence of caregivers necessitates a medicolegal framework for the treatment and rehabilitation of HMI patients. In contrast to many other marginalised groups, stigma and taboos continue to surround mental illness even today. Therefore, even when possible, the rehabilitation of those with HMI is not accepted by society. With numerous obstacles to overcome, the number of structured initiatives to serve HMI individuals in the NGO sector is significantly lower than required.

DOI: 10.4324/9781032662053-6

The Banyan, an NGO, established in 1993, is one of the first non-profit organisations that initiated a systemic venture to meet the need of the HMI persons in Chennai. Similarly, Iswar Sankalpa has been trying to serve the same purpose in Kolkata since 2007. A few more organisations have been established over the last two decades, taking the hassles and risks of being engaged with such a marginalised population. While such isolated (yet structured) ventures seem non-significant in terms of statistics, the motivation and intent behind their action matters. However small, every step towards rehabilitating an HMI person or providing them with essential resources counts. They all have faced, tackled, and are still facing the challenges that lie in the way of serving an alienated and fleeting population like the HMI persons.

As mentioned earlier, when the government's initiatives are limited, the role of the NGOs as service providers becomes crucial. The service providers are the thread that connects the rehabilitated HMI persons to mainstream society from the margin. Thus, in a study that explores the recovery and empowerment process in this population, it becomes immensely relevant to explore the motivation that helps the service providers overcome the insurmountable challenges that have been on their way.

Both NGOs have a person-centred and recovery-oriented approach toward mental health services, focusing on ensuring the holistic well-being of the service users in a dignified humane manner that may address the need for empowerment, social inclusion, and justice. Recovery, as per Dr VG, the founder and managing trustee of The Banyan, thus reverberates the following:

> Recovery depends primarily on a few conditions. First, it is self-awareness since everybody is thinking- feeling person. Thus, collaborative goal-oriented support by a few others who care can help one enhance or explore that self-awareness. Secondly, this collaborative support must be unconditional and help develop unconditional trust. Last but most important is the drive within oneself to be in command of your own life.

This recovery philosophy further gets dripped into the empowerment concept and puts its mark on it. Mrs SDR, the founder and secretary, Iswar Sankalpa, reflected:

> Empowerment gets enhanced by a meaningful relationship, but it's also about your outlook toward life. You may not have a meaningful relationship, or you may have one, but you don't consider it to be one. But what is your social world? Do you feel you have a role out there? Do you think you want to move from a state where you are taken care of to a slightly different position where you own your agency to caring for yourself and others, or do you feel there is no need to do that? So this outlook towards life is contingent not only on a meaningful

relationship but also on the environment, your social context, personality traits, past experiences, previously played social roles and interactions and the challenges and losses you have suffered. And these then would decide whether you want an empowered life or to stay dependent.

These ideological standpoints of both NGOs shaped their curriculum and have been the building block behind their actions, training service providers and ultimately having some positive effect on the end-users.

As noted in Chapter 2, the fieldwork included interviewing 20 service providers (founders, clinical psychologists, counsellors, psychiatrists, proxy caregivers, non-professional caregivers, social workers, vocational trainers, and healthcare workers) and collecting secondary data about their experiences of serving the HMI persons. An analysis of these data using the CGT approach led to the categories depicting the challenges faced by and the motivation of these service providers described in Chapter 2. The following sections thus explore the motivation and challenges experienced by the service providers from the two NGOs where I conducted my fieldwork.

The Motivation Behind Facilitating the Process of Recovery and Empowerment in HMI Persons

Social Responsibility as Intrinsic Motivation

When it comes to the factors that might motivate individuals or organisations to serve the distressed, one must be intrinsically motivated to start with. Both the founding members of The Banyan and Iswar Sankalpa highlighted this fact. Both of them had initiated their journey in their hometown (Chennai and Kolkata, respectively) since they felt that their responsibility and duty to the cities were inherently related to what they had become human beings. They felt they owed it to their cities and the people. Thus, within their limited capacity, with a dedicated team of trained and untrained individuals, they started their journey and faced the reality of the suffering of an HMI person. Mrs LR, the assistant director of Iswar Sankalpa, who had been with them since the conception of the NGO back in 2007, recollected:

> We first started having medical camps. That was the first time I came to terms with the severity of the reality of their (HMI persons) suffering. Maggot infested, malnutrition, and serious mental illness, all simultaneously. The first thing we did was to clear the maggots. It was unbelievable that a living human body could be so severely infested with maggots. That was reality. A homeless person with SMI gets shunned from everything, their reality, feelings, past, present, everything, uprooted both externally and internally. However, the beauty of the human being is that it understands love, no matter what. When we approached this

lady, she cooperated without any hesitation. The first thing that a human being responds to is love, care, and affection. The families failed in there. Before any clinical intervention, this is the first thing that they need.

Experiencing this marginalised population, irrespective of their florid symptoms and lack of insight, reacting to the love and care expressed by the service providers further reinforced their actions.

Personal Losses as Intrinsic Motivation

The founder members identified their social responsibility as the factor that initiated their journey. But for many other members who have been associated since the inception of the NGOs, it was their personal losses that motivated them to embark upon this path. For example, Mrs MM, a non-professional caregiver for Iswar Sankalpa, chose to join the NGO following the death of her husband and elder daughter.

> Before I started working with them, I had seen the death of my husband and then my twenty-two-year-old daughter. So I feel a deep emotional attachment to these girls. Some call me maa (mother), and I find the meaning of my life in them. They become so concerned and caring even if I have a fever.

Humanity as Intrinsic Motivation

For the proxy caregivers, who are not even part of the organisations directly, who are not paid for their services, and who are community members in general, this unconditional service to the distressed beings was part of their life, their humanity. For example, Mr MN, a community member and proxy caregiver with Iswar Sankalpa, run a grocery shop in Kolkata. He had cared for "Arabul" as a way of life.

> This (serving the HMI persons and the distressed) is my humanity. If I help someone, it will do good for me. But again, it is wrong if you think of your benefit when helping someone. If I earn 100 rupees, I should spend 10 rupees on someone in need. In today" s world, a son does not care for his mother. So it becomes imperative, thus, to remain humane. I have tried my best to teach this to my children and grandchildren. I hope they have internalised it and will keep practising it even when I am not there.

Whether their sense of social responsibility, humanity, or a coping mechanism against the personal losses experienced, what runs across all the service providers in The Banyan or Iswar Sankalpa, is their intrinsic motivation to serve this severely marginalised population. And this motivation, more often than usual, gets reinforced by witnessing the process of recovery and empowerment in the HMI persons to whom they provide service despite all challenges.

Challenges Experienced in Providing Service to the HMI Persons

Lack of Awareness among Stakeholders

The service providers univocally talked about the difficulty they face at the systemic level due to a lack of awareness among various stakeholders, starting with the family members, government departments, the primary healthcare system, and the community. According to Chatterjee and Das Roy (2017), associated with the Iswar Sankalpa

> The homeless and mentally ill are just a drop in the ocean of people struggling for space, services and survival in an over-burdened city. Making visible the cause of the homeless mentally ill, however vulnerable they may be, is an uphill battle in a state that ranks at the bottom of a number of socio-economic indices.
>
> (p. 767)

Lack of Existing Resources and Support at the Systemic Level

At the government level, the poor budgetary allocation towards mental health, shuffling of responsibility from one to the other department, apathy, and lack of awareness and stigma around mental illness made it challenging for the service providers at the fundamental level. Mrs CS, the shelter-in-charge of Marudyan, the male shelter house of Iswar Sankalpa, reflected:

> It has been only a systemic challenge because mental illness is the least important thing for the government. To advocate for mental illness, the amount of effort we put into all government departments, including but not exclusive to police, medical personnel, and government officials, is insurmountable. Since they are mentally ill, the Social Welfare Department pushes them to the Health Department. Because of their homelessness, Health Department shuffles them back to the Social Welfare Department.

However, the founder of The Banyan, Dr VG, had a slightly different experience. She says Tamil Nadu has a higher health indicator than other states. Moreover, the administrative system has also reacted more proactively with a better budget allocation toward mental health. She thus considers that her journey as a service provider began on a better footing than most other states.

The lack of integration of mental healthcare in the primary healthcare system has been a concern raised by researchers globally (Collins et al.,

2011). It is echoed in the experiences of the service providers as well as the challenge that it poses. Ms LR, assistant director, Iswar Sankalpa, reflected:

> Ten years down the lane, we are still fighting. The pharmacology of mental illness is hardly essential in the primary medical curriculum. The doctors are not aware. There is no support at the primary health care facilities and no awareness. Thus, even when we are rehabilitating them back to society, unless and until they are being provided medicine by us, they often discontinue the medicine again because there is no doctor to write them the medicine.

The apathy from other structured institutions like the banks also brings up newer challenges in facilitating empowerment to the HMI persons. Ms MS, who has been in charge of the vocational unit of The Banyan, highlighted the critical issues they experience because of the apathy at structural levels.

> When it comes to the homeless population, situations are different. We are struggling to get bank accounts for many of our women. They have an Aadhar card. But when we are trying to provide The Banyan address as a bona fide certificate of address proof, the bank is not accepting that. And because of that, many women have financial losses. The vocational unit is still self-sustaining. They buy raw materials, make things, and sell them and only from the profit can they provide a salary; the rest is used for repurchasing raw materials. If we had the 'bank's help, we could have initially gotten a loan for the raw materials. Their salaries could have earned some interest. We cannot have a self-help group, a corporate social group, for which we need bank accounts because it would need the details of the members' bank accounts.

Challenges in Capacity Building

Challenges at Community Level

When asked how they involve the community members to work with them, the service providers at Iswar Sankalpa identified that the community needs sensitisation. The sensitisation begins when they observe a set of dedicated workers providing for an HMI person in their locality. They witness the gradual change in that individual after being cared for, and they get motivated to become involved in the process. It is a prolonged process, but it has worked for Iswar Sankalpa almost every time. Mr TP, who has been a social worker with Iswar Sankalpa since its inception in 2007, reflected:

> Dedication on the part of the NGO is essential. You need to prove to the community that you care. For example, when we identify a homeless person on the street with SMI, we visit them every day,

even when they are paranoid and would not talk to us. Gradually he comes to understand that we will not harm him, and one day he might look at us and make eye contact, and the day he does that, the "trust" develops. The community becomes a witness to this, and they also trust us.

Challenges with the Service Users

While the large population density of Kolkata creates a massive pool for potential proxy caregivers, there also lies many challenges in rehabilitating them through the outreach programme Naya Daur (A New Run). According to Chatterjee and Das Roy (2017),

> The variables in the Naya Daur program are numerous—the incoherence of thought and emotional fragility of psychiatric patients are exacerbated by the instability of not having a roof over 'one's head, the need to scrounge for food wherever one can get it, and the transient nature of homelessness. Each street is different—some more hospitable to the homeless and mentally ill and some less so. Each patient is different. Their bonds to others in the community will be as tenuous or as trusting as her experiences in the community have been, as stable or chaotic as her current mental state. Trying to bring itinerant persons into a treatment regimen while respecting their autonomy in an unregulated space results in reduced drug compliance, dropouts from treatment, rehabilitation and supportive employment.
>
> (p. 765)

Challenges at Family Level

Even after tracing these people back to their homes, many challenges are faced by the service providers. Restitution becomes challenging, mainly because of the stigma associated with mental illness. While for men, their acceptance is not affected by their homelessness, for women, homelessness poses an additional burden of taboo. The families are counselled before the individual is reinstated, which is a slow process. Mr TP further identified some of the barriers he faced in a decade of experience in repatriating and restitution of the HMI individuals particularly women.

> The families are not often ready to take them back. They fear what others will say. They remain unsure about where the girl has been over such a long period. We insist they come over and check where she had been kept. First, we request them to take her back for a month. If things go fine, take her for another three months, then six months, and this is how we gradually expose both to each other because adjusting back is a challenge for both of them.

However, both organisations identified that reinstatement is not always an ideal solution. According to Chatterjee and Das Roy (2017),

> The restoration of persons to families and the findings on follow-up suggest a return to family is not necessarily an ideal solution. Most of the organisation's patients come from poor socio-economic back-grounds, while some are from rural areas. Some families are not equipped—either psychologically or economically—to deal with a person who has developed a mental illness, and the quality of life for the returning person does not necessarily improve…
>
> (p. 765)

Dr VG, founder of The Banyan, identified that the person often does not want to return to the family because of past experiences of dejection. And for such individuals, The Banyan has introduced their "Home Again" project, where they can live on their own terms and mimic a family-like environment within the community. For Iswar Sankalpa, "Naya Gram," an assisted community living in a village on the outskirts of Kolkata, is doing the same. The residents at Nayagram participate in agricultural work to earn their living. As a result, both the founders talk about an improved quality of life for the residents who stay there.

Intra-Institutional Hierarchy

Apart from the systemic challenges, both NGOs experience an array of intra-institutional challenges stemming from the hierarchy inbuilt into any organisational setup. Mrs LR, a clinical psychologist, associated with The Banyan for almost a decade, found it to be one of the most pressing issues.

> One of the things we try to do is an open dialogue between the workers and the service users, which is the healthiest way to resolve such issues. Before, we have tried many things for the stress they have to handle, the burn-out, etc. It's challenging to induce in every staff that the service users do not lie at the base of the hierarchy. It is for whom all of them are being employed.

Ms SA, the resident social worker with The Banyan, further identified that the mixed bag of workers, from professionals to non-professionals and community members, sometimes makes it difficult.

> Maintaining consistency amongst the workers becomes challenging because the NGO consists of professionals, non-professionals, volunteers, and interns, which becomes a mixed bag at the end of the day. However, since all of them are pro-mental health, they successfully keep providing services to these patients.

Indeed, service providers face an array of challenges which is not only dynamic but insurmountable at times. However, their immense dedication towards the service they provide in helping these alienated forgotten individuals (HMI persons) keeps them on track. And that makes them the first building blocks that initiate the process of recovery and empowerment in the HMI persons.

References

Chatterjee, D., & Roy, S. D. (2017). Iswar Sankalpa: Experience with the homeless persons with mental illness. In R.G. White, S. Jain, M. D. Orr, & U. M. Read (Eds.), *The Palgrave handbook of sociocultural perspectives on global mental health* (pp. 751–771). Palgrave Macmillan.

Collins, P. Y., Patel, V., Joestl, S. S., March, D., Insel, T. R., Daar, A. S., Bordin, I. A., Costello, E. J., Durkin, M., Fairburn, C., Glass, R. I., Hall, W., Huang, Y., Hyman, S. E., Jamison, K., Kaaya, S., Kapur, S., Kleinman, A., Ogunniyi, A., ... Walport, M. (2011). Grand challenges in global mental health. *Nature, 475*(7354), 27–30.

Patel, V., & Thara, R. (2003). Introduction: The role of NGOs in mental health care. In V. Patel & R. Thara (Eds.), *Meeting the mental health needs of developing countries: NGO innovations in India* (pp. 1–19). Sage Publications India.

7 Rehabilitation

Present Concerns and Future Directions

The individual-centric, psychopathology-oriented focus of the biomedical conceptualisation of the HMI persons limits our perception towards them solely through the disability lens. A clinical recovery orientation of the HMI persons always runs the risk of undermining the strengths and resilience of the HMI persons that may enable them to survive highly hostile environments. It becomes critically relevant to move beyond that existing discourse to recognise and make scope for their stories to be heard through their voices. A Social Constructionist paradigm with a Critical Ethnography methodology allowed me to explore those under-documented territories and consider the hierarchies that catalysed the process of becoming an HMI individual and beyond.

To recapitulate, Chapter 3 illustrated five life stories where the individuals could not go past that intense social suffering posed on their way towards recovery and empowerment but merely survived homelessness and SMI. Chapter 4 enumerated five more narratives of survivors of homelessness-SMI who had recovered and shared the experiences of empowerment to a certain extent, but due to a lack of personal or relational resources (particularly hope) impeded the process of empowerment. Chapter 5 portrayed the life stories of five individuals who survived homelessness-SMI and shared the experiences of recovery and empowerment that were closely associated with "hope." Chapter 6 explored the experience of service providers in facilitating the process of recovery and empowerment in HMI persons. This chapter explores how these representative life stories and the experiences of the service providers could address the context-based issues of rehabilitation besides the theoretical gaps in the study of the mental health experiences of HMI.

Experience of Social Suffering of HMI Individuals Associated with the Downward Mobilisation

In the book's first chapter, I highlighted the danger of medicalising a socio-economically and socio-politically constructed issue. Parallelly, it is also imperative to understand the socio-cultural and socio-historical context of the lives of HMI Individuals. Without doing so, we might overlook the

DOI: 10.4324/9781032662053-7

hierarchies and the power processes critical in mobilising them towards the margin.

In their seminal work on social suffering, Kleinman, Das, and Locke (1997) conceptualised it as the "devastating injuries" that social forces can thrust upon individuals. According to Kleinman et al. (1997), "Social suffering results from what political, economic, and institutional power does to people and, reciprocally, from how these forms of power themselves influence responses to social problems" (p. ix). In the context of HMI individuals, the framework of social suffering helps to understand the interplay of various socio-political and socio-economic forces that initiated the experience of suffering. This suffering is further aggravated by the apathy of various social institutions, including healthcare bureaucracies.

Conceptualising the socio-historical context of the vignettes' lives also helps understand how their pain and suffering did not remain limited to the individual sufferer but bled into the family and social network. Paradoxically, in the context of the life stories of these vignettes, we would also explore how suffering had been induced upon them at times within various familial-social relationships. As mentioned, looking at the problem of homelessness-cum-SMI only through the medical lens might be unwise. Social suffering as a framework helps by collapsing the categories such as healthcare, social or economic factors, or determinants (on which mental health outcomes are usually regressed using a statistics-driven biomedical model). It provides a platform to holistically understand the issues of exclusion, alienation, marginalisation, or dehumanisation within the hierarchies of class, gender, caste, religion, or geographical region. In this section, I will explain the multitude of hierarchies that have led the participants into their pathways towards homelessness and precipitated the SMI, followed by a discussion on their lived experience of homelessness and SMI.

Exclusion and Victimisation Due to Patriarchal Power Processes

Many scholars with a feminist vantage point conceptualise patriarchy as a system of social structures and practice of female subordination, oppression, and exploitation under male dominance (Walby, 1990). Goldberg (1979) described patriarchy as a system of organisation (political, economic, financial, religious, or social) where the hierarchical power positions were dominated overwhelmingly by men. The brunt of these hierarchies sustained by male dominance can be felt between two women, exercised on the son by the father, the son on the elderly parents, the boss on the employee, and likewise. Hunnicutt (2009) identified that patriarchal systems and relations exist both at the macro-level (government, bureaucracies, law, economy) and micro-level (families, communities, organisations). Indeed, gender hierarchies organise the patriarchal power processes within these levels. Still, it is mediated by race, age, class, sexuality, and religion that sustain the power distribution and privilege patterns between males and females.

In her book *We Should All Be Feminists* (2014), the Nigerian author Chimamanda Ngozi Adichie explains why evolutionarily men ruled the world since to survive the wilderness, the physically stronger of the two was more practical. However, in today's world, the same rationale is no more applicable. Today, one needs a more intelligent, knowledgeable, creative, productive, and innovative leader. Gender should not be the criteria for choosing the leader, as our "hormones" do not control leadership qualities. She regrets that though biologically, humans have evolved, our ideas of gender hardly evolved.

It is not surprising that this hierarchical power process of patriarchy would victimise a socio-economically vulnerable and alienated population. It is agonising that the HMI individuals have been victims of this process all their life; this victimisation initiated the cycle of homelessness and SMI. They have experienced dehumanisation as they have been subjected to oppression and exploitation due to the patriarchal power processes as a victim of domestic violence, denial of experience and role of motherhood, various patriarchal practices, gender-based norms, poverty, and unemployment. In the following section, I will discuss how these experiences aggravated their social suffering and initiated their downward mobilisation (a change in their position, in this case, in a downward direction towards the margins of society).

Victims of Domestic Violence

According to the World Health Organisation (WHO), domestic violence is not simply an argument. It is a pattern of coercive controls that one person exercises over another. Abusers use physical and sexual violence, threats, emotional insults and economic deprivation as a way to dominate their victims and get their way.

(as cited in Susmitha, 2016, p. 603)

Thus, it is misusing power in an intimate relationship by one adult on another person. Though domestic violence is primarily discussed in the context of gendered violence, the victims are not limited to women alone. Children, elderly parents, relatives suffering from physical or mental illness, and unemployed adults are all susceptible to being victimised by the violence within one's households.

Globally experienced across cultures, irrespective of socio-economic status, with the incidence varying from one condition to another, domestic violence is also a common phenomenon in India. However, what sets it apart in India from many other countries is the *culture of silence* engulfing it. Laws have been passed (e.g., The Protection of Women from Domestic Violence Act, 2005), committees have been formed, verdicts have been passed, and yet it continues. The life stories of the vignettes in the study reflected violence of all kinds, even within the safest of one's territories, that is, home. The participants recollected their feelings of humiliation and subjugation by familial relations through physical, emotional, and sexual abuses. Since most of my vignettes were women, their experiences might appear more pronounced; however, the male participants were equally a victim of domestic violence.

For female vignettes, the perpetrators were their parents, siblings, children, and in-laws. On the contrary, male vignettes were victimised by their siblings and cousins over property-related disputes, except for Muraad, who was disowned by his adoptive parents. However, no such pattern emerged in the experiences of the female vignettes. Instead, women are victimised because they are easy prey. Violence against women helps society to maintain unequal power distribution. There is a widespread culture of normalisation and acceptance of violence as part of marital life and male entitlement. In the equation of marriage, masculinity must dominate and control women. However, it is not necessarily the case that only the male power in the family usually subjugates, oppresses, and exploits females. For example, many males have experienced being physically tortured by their sisters-in-law or sisters, both physically and emotionally. Thus, domestic violence is more about power and control and the implicit mandate of the socio-economic context of these power relations rather than male violence that is ideologically constructed by patriarchy.

Because of the acceptance of domestic violence nurtured by its silencing culture, the reaction to abuse had primarily been flight or freeze. Hardly any of the participants fought against it. What made them get subdued? Even when abused by their in-laws, their financial dependence, concern for children's safety, lack of social support, and absence of help from other relatives, including parents, stopped Karunai or Sujaya from considering any step to be taken against their perpetrators. Damayanti, Shankar, or Lavanya chose to leave the abusive household and live independently based on financial empowerment. However, the lack of it forced Ruhi and Kavita to flee home. On the other hand, Snigdha took up prostitution to survive when she left home after years of being humiliated and dehumanised by her husband and his mother.

None of the victims considered taking any legal action against their in-laws or other perpetrators for abusing them. For most of them, domestic violence is not even a criminal offence. However, irrespective of their gender, their experience with domestic violence had a severe consequence on their life, either being the reason for becoming homeless or precipitating SMI (discussed later in respective sections).

Denial of Experience and Role of Motherhood

A significant role of females is considered to be reproduction and, thereby, Motherhood since the beginning of time. It has remained fundamental to being a "woman." It forms the base for family structure and organisation at the micro-level and the genesis of society at the macro-level. It is believed that the sexual division of labour came into the system because it was difficult for women to be mobile during the child-bearing period. Therefore, it was convenient for them to engage in domestic activities while men hunted. However, ironically, in a patriarchal society, this natural process became a means to subordinate women. In India, with a predominance of Hinduism as a religious majority, the mother goddess is worshipped in various forms throughout the nation. Maithreyi Krishnaraj (2017), in the preface to the book *Interrogating Motherhood*, points out a paradox of the social construction of motherhood in this context. On one hand, there is veneration of the mother goddess and on the other hand, deprivation of actual living mothers at the hand of patriarchy. And it is this subjugation and deprivation that the female vignettes in this study experienced as mothers at all levels – familial, social, or structural – where they have been dejected and denied the very experience of mothering their child.

Though the biological process of carrying the child in her womb for three trimesters is done by the mother, in many situations, she has no control or says in either mothering or motherhood. The female participants who were victims of child marriage (Ayesha) or were impregnated much before the legal age (Ruhi), and it took its toll on their physical and emotional health. On the contrary, Snigdha, who considered all her life that children bring happiness to a family, was forced to abort her pregnancy thrice when she wanted another child after her first two kids. After being disenchanted with her idea of a family following years of oppression, she left home and had to take up prostitution to survive. When she became pregnant, she left the profession to bring this child up. Not knowing the father's identity did not stop her mothering instincts from overlooking the societal frowns. Soon after she found a new meaning or motivation to live her life with zest as a mother, her child was taken away by the child-welfare system. The patriarchal power processes denied her rights to motherhood at all levels, familial, social, and systemic. Similarly, Karunai, Pushpavalli, or Sujaya were declared unfit to be mothers by the same socio-familial systems.

As mentioned earlier, many female vignettes never dared to stand against their perpetrators to protect their children. As mothers, they were concerned that since they were financially dependent on the family, they would be unable to look after their children if they spoke up against domestic violence. Damayanti, who was financially empowered, chose to leave her husband to protect her child and give him the life she believed he deserved. Many were forced to give up their rights and custody of their children when they got diagnosed with SMI (discussed later).

Because of this overwhelming control of the patriarchal power process in every aspect of motherhood and mothering, Krishnaraj (2017) laments how the function of motherhood lies in maintaining patriarchy, "Motherhood actual contribution is to maintain patriarchy: the dominance of the male through the triple instruments of control over reproduction, sexuality and sexual division of labour" (para. 8).

Being a Victim of Patriarchal Practices

The female participants talked about feeling exploited and suffocated as victims of cultural norms initiated and maintained by patriarchal practices. It included but was not exclusive to child marriage, the responsibility to sustain male lineage, widowhood, the standard of feminine beauty, etc. The cultural expectation of Indian women to be chaste and obedient moulds them into accepting these prescribed gender roles. However, their approval of this role does not necessarily mean their appreciation; rather, it represents the tolerance they develop through lifelong training in assuming the role of an ideal Indian woman.

The emergence of a patriarchal hierarchy can be traced throughout the foundations of India's history, so profoundly rooted that even today, we let the malpractices of patriarchy continue in the name of culture and heritage. Despite the existing laws against it, child marriage is still rampant in various parts of the country, mainly among the lower socio-economic status (SES) families of rural India. Many vignettes, who were from such a background, became victims of child marriage. It is hardly a custom in Indian families from such a background to seek the girl's consent before marrying them off. Thus, without understanding the complexities of marriage, the dynamics of leaving their parents, living in a new household, and adjusting to different circumstances, Ayesha got married to a fellow pavement dweller when she was ten years old.

Widowhood, in India, is another means of female subordination and oppression against their rights to property, social status, and empowerment. Even with the law on their side, once widowed, the individual becomes a non-entity for the in-laws and a burden to the parents and siblings even today. The situation of Indian widows for centuries evolved through the demolition of Sati and the introduction of the Hindu Widows remarriage Act of 1856; a lot of their suffering remains unnoticed even today. However, with little representation in policies, neglected and invisible, they are still abused and violated even in 21st-century India (Sahoo, 2014). Given that, when Pushpavalli's husband committed suicide following an argument with her maternal relatives, she considered herself responsible for his death. The blames received from her in-laws only enhanced the guilt and grief. Eight months pregnant then, she was not even allowed back to her in-law's place following her husband's death. She ultimately ended up at The Banyan when her mother failed to provide for her treatment for SMI.

Patriarchy also entails initiating and maintaining norms for standardising feminine and masculine qualities. While "fair and lovely" formed the parameter for women's beauty, "rough and tough" set the standard for masculinity. Within the social contours of caste, class, community, and marriage circles, fair-skin colour, and other feminine embellishments accentuate marital, caste, and class positions and validate feminine gender identity. Fairer skin is further a commentary on unmarried females' moral, behavioural, and cultural chastity. Thus, despite having the same educational qualification as her younger sister and being financially empowered, because of being dark, Kavita never got married. Families after families of potential grooms scrutinised her in the parameters set by the patriarchal norms and chose to reject her. This made her believe that her worth was based on the complexion of her skin. And it is well established how an unmarried daughter of marriageable age might become a burden even to her parents. Deprived of her wish and will, when her parents gave up on her, Kavita too tried to bury in vain her dream to have a family of her own, to get married and become a mother. These rejection and humiliation experiences added to her baggage of cumulative stressors that eventually precipitated the SMI.

Being a Victim of Exploitation Based on Gender Norms

V. Geetha (2002), in her book, *Gender*, delineates,

> Gender is everywhere. When we dress a girl child in soft colours and frilly clothes, buy a male child a gun, when we admonish girls for behaving like boys, or tease boys being timid 'like girls', we are 'doing' gender. That is, we are allocating to the male and female sexes specific and distinctive attributes and roles; likewise, we also impose different sets of expectations on them.
>
> (p. xiii)

Thus, when Karunai was made to leave school after the fourth standard, she did not find anything unusual, for that was the norm. She rationalised that the girls should stay home and engage in household chores. Similarly, even when she was a diligent student, Kavita was forced to leave school after the tenth standard with the same rationale. She was also forced to leave the job she did since it was not appreciated in her society.

The United Nation's declaration on the Elimination of Violence Against Women (1993) defines violence against women as: "... any act of gender-based violence that results in, or is likely to result in, physical, sexual or psychological harm or suffering to women" (p. 2). Apart from being abused physically and emotionally at a domestic level, many female vignettes talked about their experiences of being sexually exploited before they had the same experience as homeless women. For most, these experiences started within the protective walls of their own home by their relatives. The feeling of dehumanisation experienced due to being sexually violated bore a long-term significance in their life beyond being affected by homelessness or SMI. Many of them considered it challenging to stay independently outside the realm of the shelter houses owing to their past experiences or for considering themselves vulnerable based on the "gender norms."

Being a Victim of Poverty and Unemployment

As it reverberated across their life stories, most participants, even before homelessness, belonged to a lower socio-economic status. While homelessness is one of the extreme outcomes of poverty, it has a strong foothold in every other aspect of an individual's life, including the onset and maintenance of mental illness. Poverty is one of the main contributing factors to poor living conditions and lack of adequate housing, education, sanitation, and nutrition, resulting in poor health conditions, both physical and psychological. The poor cannot afford to stay ill since they mainly survive on their daily wages. Thus, they spend out of pocket to meet their treatment need, which worsens due to lack of access to adequate resources, including treatment facilities, leading further to stress, deteriorating quality of life, and diminished well-being, which again keeps them stuck in the poverty-ill health nexus.

The vignettes, in their childhood, were rendered deprived because of their parents' resourcelessness. This affected their education which reduced their chances of employability in future. Thus, some of them, particularly the males, found themselves stuck in menial jobs as adults. While the female vignettes were not socially expected to earn their livelihoods, the male participants expressed their agony and humiliation at being unemployed or lowly paid. Because they were not making enough, the male participants felt "inadequate" socially and were also victims of domestic violence. When unemployed, Pradeepto started abusing alcohol, and instead of receiving help, he was beaten and rendered homeless by his relatives. The male members of the family who are unable to earn and be financially empowered are considered a burden to the system, both familial and social, and may often become victims of domestic violence.

The experiences of dehumanisation of the vignettes provide some insights into how the interplay of various familial and social processes guided by patriarchal power practices and gender norms initiated social suffering. The following section will portray the vignettes' experiences with patriarchal power processes that led them towards the pathway to homelessness or contributed to precipitating the SMI.

The Lived Experiences of Homelessness among HMI Individuals

Meaning of Home and Homelessness

Reiterating from the first chapter, the operational definition of home as conceived by Aashray Adhikar Abhiyan (AAA) to contextualise homelessness is

> [one] who has no place to call home in the city. By home is meant a place which not only provides a shelter but takes care of one's health, social, cultural and economic needs. Home offers a holistic care and security (sic).
>
> (as cited in Tipple & Speak, 2005, p. 347)

This definition, which is extensive and holistic enough to accommodate the essential social and emotional factors to make a shelter adequate to become a home, has moved much beyond the classical accommodation-oriented approach to defining home. It also echoed the meaning of home that the vignettes found for themselves. Home, for them, is a space that might provide independent agency to access resources, where one is settled and rooted with "loved ones" and is being mutually cared for. On the contrary, homelessness was perceived as being uprooted without happiness, peace, and comfort in the company of loved ones.

Some vignettes could perceive the shelter houses as home. However, it was more challenging for others to understand the shelter house as anything more than a temporary solution. The essence of being cared for and the experience of happiness became prominent in their meaning of home for Chethana or Sujaya, who were forced to leave "homes." Many vignettes could perceive the shelter or shared houses as their home. On the contrary, for Damayanti, who was homeless as a consequence of SMI, or Snigdha, who had significant and meaningful relations outside the shelter houses, it was challenging to consider the shelter houses as home as they looked forward to a life outside the shelter house, or with their families, especially their children.

Suffering Associated with Homelessness

Life on the streets is meant to be harsh. Apart from suffering from a lack of shelter, food, and clothing, that is all the necessary amenities of life, the vignettes suffered through extreme dehumanisation and humiliation by being physically, sexually, and emotionally tormented due to being vulnerable as homeless. Moreover, as most participants were actively symptomatic during their stay on the streets, they could not protect themselves in most scenarios.

The vignettes recollected their experiences of physical assaults where they lost all their possessions to the goons. In addition, they remembered being teased, taunted, and sometimes beaten by community members or harassed by police. It is beyond doubt that these experiences exacerbated the social suffering of the participants. While none of the male vignettes opened up about being sexually assaulted on the streets (given that I was of the opposite gender and there is a lower rate of disclosure of males being sexually abused), it was one of the most common traumas that the female vignettes suffered while living on the streets.

The dehumanisation experienced by the women on the streets due to sexual assaults ranged from being molested and raped on multiple occasions, being impregnated because of rape, becoming a victim of human trafficking, and being forced into prostitution. While Ruhi fled home to escape the sexual assault at home, on the streets, she had been raped by community members and police personnel and had become pregnant. She had also been trafficked across the border from Bangladesh to India and forced into prostitution. In addition, many female vignettes reported being assaulted sexually by police personnel towards whom they had turned for safety when they (female vignettes) sensed being vulnerable. The breach of trust they had experienced at home thus continued even when homeless and vulnerable.

Interestingly the experience of sexual exploitation was reported by women who ended up on the streets in the eastern or northern parts of India. Not a single woman who remained homeless within the South Indian states reported being sexually assaulted on the streets. It does corroborate with the reports of the National Crime Records Bureau that show much lesser crime against women, including rape and molestation, in states like Tamil Nadu or Karnataka (West Bengal 69.1; Tamil Nadu 8.6; Crime in India 2021 Statistics Volume 1, p. 221). According to their report, in 2021, Tamil Nadu reported 1.1 rape cases in contrast to West Bengal's rate of 2.3 (Crime in India – 2018 Statistics Volume 1, 2020, p. 218).

Surviving Homelessness

As mentioned earlier, life on the streets lacked all the fundamental amenities needed to survive. Nevertheless, the participants survived both homelessness and SMI and myriads of physical, sexual, and emotional assaults. They shared that the demands of living on the streets compelled them to learn strategies (like identifying safe zones and food providers) to survive homelessness. In social science, there has seldom been a concern about how HMI individuals survive the inordinately hostile environments or what creative strategies they use. Instead, the focus has remained generally confined to understanding them through a "disability" lens.

Many female vignettes identified that staying within the compound of a temple would help them in multiple ways. They got their two times meals from the "prasadam" (food that had been offered to the deity and later distributed among devotees). It also provided them with a safe shelter from the goons outside. Many of them reported identifying food shops that would give them food. For Bijon and Shankar, such community involvement helped the social workers identify their proxy caregivers. The female vignettes also recollected that when they stayed among a crowd, they felt safer than staying alone, where there was always the risk of being assaulted. Staying hyper-vigilant, scanning the environment, and avoiding dangerous places helped many vignettes survive on the streets. Even when homeless, Shankar had managed to bag himself a job and continued doing it even after the onset of SMI until he was seriously injured in a traffic accident.

With the focus of the policymakers on what is wrong with this marginalised population, we often end up overlooking what is right with them. The zeal to survive the insurmountable hurdles is one of the driving forces that led them to return to the mainstream of life in the community from the shelter homes. However, that alone would not be enough until the responsible stakeholders identify their responsibilities towards them and execute them.

The Lived Experiences of SMI among HMI Individuals

Meaning Making of Symptoms and Suffering Associated with SMI

The overwhelming experiences of life-long struggle against pervasive losses and dehumanisation often left the vignettes with one question: "Why did the illness happen?" Asking the question is an essential step towards "meaning making." Meaning making is a pervasive, enduring, but dynamic feeling that the world is comprehensible. It helps in believing that future challenges are manageable and that efforts to overcome those challenges are meaningful and worthwhile. It is critical for recovery. While many participants could not get an answer to "Why did the illness happen?" some managed to gain some clarity. They developed meaning through the existing belief system, identifying stressful life events, behaviour, or thoughts that precipitated the illness.

Many vignettes like Sujaya, and Lavanya believed that they had been victims of someone doing "black magic" on them, making them "ill." It is not that they identified that to be the only reason. Like many other vignettes, they, too, identified significant stressful life events, trauma, and pervasive losses as a precipitator of their mental illness. The male participants identified that job loss and unemployment significantly pushed them towards poverty, homelessness, and, ultimately, SMI. The social causation-social drift theories have long advocated poverty being a causal and maintenance factor of schizophrenia (Lund, 2014; Read, 2010). Following job loss or homelessness, for some vignettes like Pradeepto and Muraad, substance abuse made it more challenging to come out of the vicious loop.

Across the vignettes' gender, domestic violence was reported as a significant precipitator. Violence of all forms against women is already an established causal factor for SMI globally by various feminist theorists and WHO (Kumar et al., 2013). However, with the focus on violence against women, feminist theories of violence struggle to understand the violence experienced by men and, in particular, the elevated risk of violence experienced by men with mental disorders (Khalifeh & Dean, 2010). Death of significant others, particularly primary caregivers, played an important role as a stressor on some participants like Chethana (parents' death), Damayanti (mother's death), Sujaya (mother-in-law's death), and Pushpavalli (husband's suicide). Their relationship with these significant others was one of their most meaningful bonds, and the sudden withdrawal of that support system created a vacuum they were unprepared for. The absence of other meaningful relationships that could have helped them redevelop their social support made the participants further vulnerable.

Double Jeopardy of "Being Unaware of" and "Apathetic Nature" of
Service Provision

The vignettes with the history of onset of SMI while at home often reported experiencing the distress of "being uncared for" due to service providers' lack of awareness, apathy, and negligence. At times, it was not that their primary caregivers were not caring enough to provide them with the required resources. But, the lack of awareness about mental disorders made it difficult for them to understand the signs of SMI. While for many participants like Damayanti or Lavanya, the "prodromal phases"[1] remained unnoticed till the onset of the psychosis, or worse, till they left home during the symptomatic phase. As the signs appeared, some vignettes were taken to faith healers or general physicians. However, for most of them, non-adherence due to caregivers' apathy and non-compliance due to their own lack of awareness disrupted the pharmacological treatment even if it was started. This almost always resulted in multiple relapses.

Apathy and negligence of the service providers within the healthcare system further exacerbated the social suffering of the vignettes. When Damayanti left home for the first time, though her brother took her to a general physician, she never got treatment since the doctor made no diagnosis at that time. Inadequate information or misinformation received from the physicians may increase their emotional distress. Thus, the unawareness about mental illness and the line of treatment in the primary healthcare system, apart from the apathy and negligence of the treating physicians, bore some significant consequences on these vignettes' lives.

Consequences of Suffering SMI

Echoed through all the participants' life stories were their experiences of being dehumanised and deprived due to the brunt of losses and stigma associated with SMI. The vignettes reflected on their feelings of being ignored and dejected on experiencing the multifaceted losses related to suffering SMI and an extreme form of social alienation and marginalisation due to the stigmatised identity of being mentally ill.

The participants expressed their suffering from losing "stability" and "normalcy" due to the illness. Damayanti and Kavita talked about missing out on the "normalcy" of life's course. Muraad found it challenging to relate to mainstream society after years of disconnection and alienation.

The vignettes recollected their feeling of being immensely betrayed, dejected, or guilty of losing significant relationships or being denied their rights to shelter, treatment, and care by the family members. Most participants reflected on being betrayed by their primary caregivers, including but not exclusive of siblings, husbands, in-laws, and children. This feeling of betrayal and dejection stemmed from their relatives failing to provide them with their fundamental rights of shelter, care, and treatment. Once diagnosed or when the signs of the illness started appearing, they were considered "burden." Nalini talked about the helplessness of their caregivers because of their resourcelessness in being unable to shelter them. However, vignettes like Chethana, Karunai, Damayanti, and Snigdha once again became victims of the all-pervading patriarchal power process and stigma associated with mental illness. The shelter was denied to them when the NGOs attempted restitution following their homelessness. In a society like India, where women's chastity and purity are so critical, it is unacceptable for women to wander the streets as a socio-moral norm. Hence, homeless women are invisible, and in the case of those with mental illness who have wandered for a period, the family rarely accepts them back home. Karunai and Chethana remembered being rejected by their relatives when they returned home after a period of homelessness, questioning their "characters" on moral grounds.

While the caregivers failed in their responsibilities towards the participants, they (vignettes) also felt overwhelming guilt for failing their relatives, primarily as mothers. Pushpavalli and Sujaya were made to understand they were "unfit" mothers to take care of their newborns, and the babies would be better off if they were given up for adoption. Pushpavalli regretted her decision retrospectively, though Sujaya still thought she had neither the means nor the ability to provide for her daughter. Ruhi, too, had given up her child for adoption. On considering herself resourceless, the teenage homeless mother decided to give her daughter up for adoption.

On the other hand, Snigdha's daughter was taken from her by the state since they deemed her to be an "unfit" mother. Her hope to be reunited with her daughter once again kept Snigdha fighting against all the odds. Karunai lamented failing in her responsibilities towards her children and families owing to their illnesses.

The participants highlighted feeling rejected, helpless, and worthless on the loss of opportunity, employment, and access to resources following SMI. Damayanti, who had left home in the symptomatic phase with all her documents related to bank, life insurance, and pension, lost them all while she was on the streets. The loss not only affected her financial well-being but also caused her significant emotional distress due to the uncertainty it created for her future. Muraad left his training as a doctor unfinished because of the cumulative stressors that ultimately precipitated the illness. Later, when he tried to enrol back in the course, he was not allowed due to red tape. As a result, he lost his opportunity to be financially empowered and independent and have a resourceful life to his mental health condition.

Bijon reflected on the fact that because of his illness, he would never be able to start a family of his own, as no one would like to marry a person with a mental illness. After years of oppression, now a victim of self-stigmatisation, he considered himself not worthy of any job of responsibility. He also lost any prospect of a better future.

Even when clinically recovered, Chethana identified that it was complicated to move beyond the stigmatised identity of being mentally ill. Even when she wanted to move beyond, the system would not let her. Lavanya recollected similar experiences. She felt losing her agency and autonomy once the label of mental illness was issued following her first-time hospitalisation. It not only took a toll on her self-esteem but also made it difficult for her to continue in the same job. She lost multiple jobs once her diagnosis came to the fore, overshadowing all her other identities and leaving her with the identity of being a patient. While Lavanya gave up on her hope that there would be any different identity for her beyond that of a "patient," Chethana looked forward to when society would accept her for her abilities, looking beyond her mental illness.

In a neoliberal society with an increased focus on individual responsibility and limited accountability of the state, it thus makes one question, where exactly do we stand as a community when the state washes the hands off the responsibility. The policies fail in their purposes to serve those for whom they were meant to be. To keep pace with the neoliberal policies, when India revised her existing mental health act in 2017, it failed to capture the disabling aspects of familial, societal, and attitudinal barriers despite the UNCRPD's attempts to shift the policy's gaze towards a social paradigm.

Thus far, we have explored how social suffering pervades all dimensions of the life of HMI individuals through the familial, societal, systemic, and structural barriers to having the experience of well-being or mental health. The extreme forms of social alienation and exclusion that they experience as a marginalised population make it even more difficult for them to overcome because of the neoliberal globalisation era that commodifies human abilities, skills, or experiences of mental health as marketable products (Bhatia & Priya; 2018; Mills, 2018). Charmaz (2020) posited that "Dominant perspectives, policies, and practices affect experiencing stigma and exclusion" (p. 21). In the following section, I would thus explore the challenges they experience towards recovery and empowerment while placed in this era of neoliberal globalisation.

Challenges towards Recovery and Empowerment

It has long been a concern that the "marginalised sections" of society, such as the HMI individuals, are denied their voices in determining their life course and establishing their identity in the name of the greater common good. For centuries, the *powerful*, rather than the vulnerable, have decided what would be "good" for it. Thus, in a society ruled by men, women become marginalised. In a world designed by the "able-bodied," "disabilities" are sectionalised, or where heterosexuality is the norm, homosexuality gets frowned upon or discriminated against. The discourse popularised by the powerful has remained the dominant discourse that excludes the alternate discourses to the margins.

In a neoliberal society, all service approaches conceptualise the individual as the "consumer," which is highly ironical for any marginalised or alienated population. And, such superimposed *individualised responsibility* for "illness," "recovery," or "empowerment" disguised as "voice," "freedom', or "agency" runs the risk of amplifying the existing social suffering further for a population like HMI individuals as they end up fighting for services, welfare, and amenities (Sharma & Priya, 2020).

This section attempts to understand the challenges towards recovery and empowerment as experienced by the HMI persons. The challenges they encounter against the dominant discourse in a neoliberal society as marginalised individuals would be discussed along with those that the service-providers experience at systemic and structural levels.

Conditions of Inaccessibility to Resources Related to Socio-economic and Community-Based Constraints

As discussed earlier, the lack or inaccessibility of essential socio-economic resources often intensified the existing suffering experienced by the vignettes. However, even when provided with shelter and treatment for the mental illness, those challenges (the brunt of patriarchal power processes, poverty, unemployment, etc.) persisted in their lives, albeit in a different form, impeding their growth towards recovery and empowerment.

A marginalised population like HMI persons often depend on the state and community to bring a change in their social position (upward mobilisation) towards a more socially integrated life where they may gain access and control over valued social resources. However, in a nation where their citizenship is often debated (e.g., the recent Citizenship Amendment Act, 2019), some of them might not have the identity proofs that the government would require. Moreover, the unavailability of Aadhaar (a 12-digit unique identity number for residents or passport holders of India based on their biometric and demographic data, including a permanent address) stops them from availing of a lot of facilities and schemes introduced to facilitate the poor and unemployed ("How will the homeless citizens get Aadhaar? SC asks Government," 2018).

The service providers in the NGOs have experienced difficulty at systemic and structural levels due to the lack of awareness among various stakeholders, be it family members, government institutions, the primary healthcare system, or the community. While Indian families have a high threshold of acceptance for the "physically ill" in the family, the situation changes rampantly when it comes to individuals diagnosed with mental illness, particularly women. Lack of awareness, the taboo about homelessness, and the stigma around mental illness force families to deny the necessary care, shelter, and acceptance that this population deserve. Thus, reinstatement does not work well in many situations, even when the families could be traced back following homelessness. Economically or emotionally unequipped, the families are often helpless – Pushpavalli and her sister were left to stay at the shelter house by their ageing and financially underprivileged parents. Often, it has been observed that when the parents die, other family members refuse to shoulder any further responsibility, as Chethana, Sujaya, Damayanti, and Pradeepto were refused shelter and care by brothers, cousins, or uncles following the death of their parents or primary caregivers and then, there are situations where the families wilfully "dump" the person in a shelter home or refuse access back at home. With almost no possibility of returning home, they are forced to stay at the shelter houses provided by the NGOs.

Though provided with shelter by the NGO (which is not a "home" for many), the lack of a steady income, a permanent job, or the absence of necessary documents makes their helplessness more pronounced. Moreover, poor budgetary allocation (less than one rupee per capita), shuffling responsibilities from one department to another, and apathy around this population have often kept the government or policymakers from providing schemes that might facilitate the HMI persons' journey towards the mainstream. Further, the absence of an inclusive attitude of other stakeholders, like the banks, also brings up newer challenges like opening a bank account for the HMI individuals, getting loans to buy raw materials for the vocational units at the NGOs, or forming corporate social groups.

At the community level, the service providers also experience difficulties facilitating community-based rehabilitation for a population such as HMI individuals. HMI persons require mental illness treatment, but poor awareness, apathy, and stigma related to mental illness make it an immense challenge for the service providers. The community often identifies a homeless person with SMI as a "nuisance" or "menace". Thus, instead of letting the person remain on the street while being treated, *community members almost always ask service providers to "take them away" from that locality.*

However, Iswar Sankalpa identified that their unique programme, *Naya Daur* (new era), had helped them greatly sensitise the community and develop a massive pool of proxy caregivers on the streets of Kolkata by slowly and gradually involving the community. Though Naya Daur has greatly improved the quality of life of the individuals involved (discussed in the section "Process of Recovery and Empowerment"), the risks involved could not be overlooked. As identified by the service providers from Iswar Sankalpa, significant variability is the "transient" nature of this population, making it challenging to keep track of them as they keep moving from one area to the other. The symptoms of SMI make this struggle all the more difficult. Even when rehabilitated into the community, the individuals prefer to stay in that "street corner" which has been "home" for them (Ayesha lived at the same street corner ever since she was a child). And this maintains their vulnerability that ranges from daily neglect and hunger to health problems, sexual abuses, and victimisation to crime (Bijon and Shankar getting harassed by local goons) besides proneness to substance abuse. The community care model also falls short during these extreme vulnerabilities (Ayesha's death due to a lack of timely medical intervention) for persons addicted to drugs or those with a severe co-morbid physical illness such as tuberculosis or HIV/AIDS.

The absence of adequate social support beyond the service providers becomes a massive challenge for many participants, particularly women and the elderly. Most women found it unacceptable to go out and live independently outside the safe wall of the shelter house without a "man to protect" them from all the dangers. With a 64.5% reported rate of Crime against Women per one lakh population of women in India (National Crime Records Bureau, 2021), women often sense threat to their safety. However, within this apprehension also lies the embedded meaning of *normalising* gender-based violence. Women's subjugation and gender hierarchies are established, promoted, and maintained implicitly within the garb of everyday realities of patriarchal practices.

Ageing-related physical ailments and the associated helplessness due to the lack of adequate social support make it extremely difficult for elderly HMI persons to live independently while undertaking any new venture outside the NGO. Furthermore, persons with SMI have a life expectancy of 25 years shorter than the general population, with a higher vulnerability to cardiovascular diseases and other health problems (National Association of State Mental Health Program Directors, 2006, as cited in Shibusawa & Padgett, 2009). Because they have no one else to look after them outside the shelter houses, even empowered and recovered women like Damayanti had been reluctant to move outside the shelter house when her brother denied her shelter but remained dependent on the NGO.

Conditions of Inaccessibility to Resources Related to Motivational Constraints

Being hopeful about their future has been the driving force for the participants towards recovery and empowerment. In contrast, hopelessness has impeded this transition (elaborated in a subsequent section). Participants have shared how they find it challenging to move outside the vigilance of the NGO when it comes to taking responsibility for their medication. Many of them (Karunai, Pushpavalli, and Nalini) found it challenging to adhere to their treatment regime when they were on their own; many a time, the auditory hallucinations or paranoid delusions "controlling" them and "stopping" them from continuing the medicine. Thus, they preferred the status quo rather than considering newer challenges to overcome.

With chronic SMI, social alienation, and seclusion, the ageing participants also found it difficult to relate to mainstream society. Muraad struggled with feeling out of sync with their "normal" peers. Some attribute this feeling to the intense deprivation of homelessness and accompanying survival mechanisms. Further, the negative experience of stigmatisation both caused and intensified the feelings of not being "normal." For the ageing population (Muraad, Pushpavalli, Damayanti), awareness of one's age sometimes heightened these feelings.

Thus, due to the adverse conditions, it becomes generally difficult for HMI persons to remain motivated and hopeful about their life in the immediate future or what the future entails for them. More specifically, the elderlies preferred to maintain the "present stability" in most situations. While such a stand sustains the symptom amelioration, it slows down or hinders the journey towards recovery and empowerment.

Consequences of Being Dependent on the NGO

Equivocally all the participants acknowledged the aid they received from the two NGOs. The critical role that the mental health community played in facilitating the recovery and empowerment of the HMI persons will be discussed in a subsequent section. However, some participants expressed feeling humiliated, unheard, and uncared for within the hierarchical system of these NGOs. These feelings are apparently associated with a lack of space for voice and independence due to the intra-institutional hierarchies. Lang (2000) has expressed his concern about whether NGOs could effectively promote and practice "democracy" within their organisations and if the failure to do so makes them less effective in their purpose.

While the working philosophy for both NGOs is engrained in a person-centred and recovery-oriented approach ensuring holistic well-being to the service users in a dignified, humane manner, the intra-institution hierarchies and inadequate efforts towards democratic functioning within the organisation may not help realise this philosophy. Participants reported how they were answerable to the service providers for every decision they made, no matter how petty they were. At times, they experienced that generalised decisions taken by the service providers were imposed upon them without being concerned about their "feelings." For example, Damayanti could not have a cup of a health drink when she wanted because it was not "allowed." They also felt belittled due to their accountability for financial transactions. Ruhi expressed her exasperation at being questioned every time she asked for even ten rupees from her account.

Furthermore, the participants often found it disagreeable to stay amidst other "symptomatic co-residents" as it interfered with their well-being. While some reported being attacked by a co-resident, others talked about having difficulty coping with those who were still "mad" (perceived as such due to poor hygiene or disorganised behaviours). Despite being sympathetic towards their co-residents, they expressed a genuine concern and were even seconded by their service providers. However, the poor infrastructure, lack of adequate human and financial resources, and absence of sufficient government support kept the service providers from providing shared housing (like the "Home Again" project of The Banyan) to all clinically recovered residents.

Even when they were aware of all the positive impact the NGOs had in their lives, these inconsequential incidents played havoc in their way towards recovery and empowerment, especially the lack of compassion and respect and the demeaning attitudes of some stakeholders. Moreover, such adverse structural factors were often associated with stigmatisation, which, in turn, affected the individuals' resources for coping. Among such negative aspects were the increased social alienation, the invasion of one's dignity, and the reduced prospect of help-seeking.

A sense of rebuilding selfhood might be facilitative towards rehabilitation. But when socially alienated and marginalised individuals felt that their independence had been restrained and their voices had been suppressed, redeveloping that sense of selfhood often decelerates. In the following section, I will discuss the multitude of ways the participants approached their resurgence from the downward mobilisation and marginalisation they experienced.

The Process of Recovery and Empowerment

In the article titled "Recovery as a Journey of the Heart," Patricia Deegan posited that the ultimate goal of recovery is not to attend normality. Instead, "The goal is to embrace the human vocation of becoming more deeply, more fully human" (Deegan, 1996, p. 92). By the clinical recovery standard, very few individuals with SMI would recover completely. However, the recovery-based mental health services for SMI have come a long way from conceptualising "clinical recovery" as the sole purpose. Instead, reconceptualising recovery through a *personal* and *existential* lens over the existing clinical and social perspective, the "recovery movement" has established recovery as a process that is "personally empowering, raising realistic hope for a better life alongside whatever remains of illness and vulnerability" (Robert & Wolfson, 2004, p. 37).

As discussed in Chapter 1, recovery is an intensely personal process, an attitude, and a way of life. Anthony (1993, Anthony et al., 2002) has emphasised that a recovery-oriented mental health service approach needs to include what the individuals who have recovered from SMI found *useful*. However, what standard textbooks in psychiatry preach is far from what one needs. On the contrary, anthologies of personal and self-evaluated accounts of individuals accommodating their illness and recovering around it have remained core to the "recovery movement."

While recovery has been designated as a personal process, empowerment is understood as a community-involved process "through which people lacking an equal share of valued resources gain greater access to and control over those resources" (Cornell University Empowerment Group, 1989, as cited in Zimmerman, 2000, p.43). In the recovery-based mental health service approaches, empowerment has been coupled with recovery forming two central pillars for holistic psychiatric rehabilitation. Psychiatric rehabilitation is "giving people with psychiatric disabilities the opportunity to work, live in the community, and enjoy a social life, at their own pace, through planned experiences in a respectful, supportive, and realistic atmosphere" (Rutman, 1993, p. 1, as cited in Corrigan et al., 2008, p. 51).

In the following segment, I will discuss how "hope" evolved as an anchor and guide to the participants' journey towards recovery and empowerment, despite social suffering or challenges experienced by them. In this context, the development and mending of social ties and how they facilitated access to valued social resources for the present participants will be discussed. In the final segment, I would elaborate on how selfhood as a fundamental aspect of recovery also becomes critical for empowerment in HMI individuals.

Trajectories of Hope in Shaping the Process of Recovery and Empowerment

As a component integral to recovery and empowerment, hope is considered a trigger and a maintaining factor for individuals with SMI. It is "hope" that initiates the journey towards recovery and empowerment and keeps them going. However, nurturing hope to begin the process of recovery and empowerment is more complicated than one can presume. With no or reduced expectations and responsibilities from self and society, SMI induces a state of learned helplessness, making it more difficult for them to generate hope.

For a marginalised population like HMI persons, burdened with the double jeopardy of homelessness and SMI, garnering hope becomes more critical yet necessary for recovery and empowerment. While I witnessed a few participants sharing their experience of hope with me, it was heart-wrenching to see others live a bleak grey with no hope to foster. Therefore, considering the frameworks of recovery and empowerment mentioned earlier, I would elaborate on how hope may shape these processes among the HMI persons.

The Broken Ties and The Lost Hopes

In Chapter 3, I illustrated the life stories of Ruhi, Kavita, Lavanya, Muraad, and Nalini. Social suffering entails "devastating injuries" that can be "overpowering" or overwhelming (Charmaz, 2002, p. 310); it might have deprived them of the streaks of hopefulness that could have guided them further towards recovery and empowerment. To understand what was making it so challenging for them to nurture hope to overpower the hurdles of the lived experiences of homelessness and SMI, the *absence of significant social ties* in all these stories became apparent.

While the ability to form and maintain social ties is critical in social interaction and positive health outcomes in SMI, it is not unusual for individuals with SMI, particularly those with experiences of homelessness, to struggle with developing social ties (Padgett et al., 2008). Pahwa et al. (2019) reported that formerly homeless individuals with SMI found it challenging to create new social ties owing to many factors that interfered with forming or maintaining connections or socialising. For example, it could be related to stigma, symptoms of mental illness and death or loss of significant others.

The participants whose life stories were presented in Chapter 3 experienced the loss of or estrangement from family relationships. While Ruhi, Kavita, and Lavanya chose to abandon their families of origin because of the life-long humiliation and dehumanisation enforced by the patriarchal power processes, Muraad became a victim when his adoptive parents disowned him. However, the helplessness of Nalini's family forced them to leave their two daughters diagnosed with SMI at the NGO. In addition, the overwhelming burden of caregiving for their children diagnosed with SMI, poverty and later, their old age got in their way. For Nalini and Lavanya, some of their biochemical treatment-resistant symptoms made it challenging to develop and maintain meaningful social ties.

Culturally alienated and far from their homelands, Ruhi in a different country, and Kavita in a socio-culturally different state from her own, it was all the way more difficult for them to find a cultural space for themselves where some meaningful social ties could be developed. Furthermore, language differences also became a barrier to developing such relational bonds for many individuals. For example, owing to the language difference in a new socio-cultural setup, Kavita could not share her thoughts or feelings for months with anyone until she met me.

Muraad, Nalini, and Lavanya might have also found their advancing age interfering with their motivation to initiate social ties. Shibusawa and Padgett (2009) reported that the insights developed with the awareness of their age in numbers, elderly HMI persons often perceived their lives through the losses they had incurred all their life and regretted their past. This might exacerbate the already existing poor motivation among elderly HMI persons. Furthermore, as Muraad reflected, having difficulty reconnecting with mainstream society interfered with their motivation to rekindle the lost social relations. Similarly, the futility of their suffering with no one to look forward to make their future appears all the more desolate.

While persons with SMI have a lower life expectancy than their counterparts, it was unknown whether the elderly HMI participants were aware of it. Nevertheless, Nalini explicitly expressed her awareness of the "time left." One of the more intriguing gerontological theories about awareness of *time left* is the socioemotional selectivity theory proposed by Carstensen et al. (1999). It states that "perceptions of limited 'time left' prompt older individuals to find emotional meaning from life as opposed to seeking out new experiences" (as cited in Shibusawa & Padgett, 2009, p. 94). Nalini further exclaimed, seeing a sense of serenity and recluse in offering herself and her future at the mercy of her God, knowing to herself that only death would bring her independence and joy against all earthly sufferings. However, the effect of cumulative adversities left them with little or no motivation to explore a potentially more meaningful future. Having far less *time left* and a deeply uncertain future, the lingering effects of long-term deprivation and repeated victimisation left the elderly HMI persons far more alienated. Nevertheless, they somehow adapted to the status quo in their struggle with social isolation and exclusion.

It is apparent from their narratives that all five stories mentioned in Chapter 3 experienced overwhelming effects of social suffering that included estrangement from their family relationships. Therefore, they found it challenging to develop social ties. If we go back to their life stories, it would not be surprising to see that all of them had experienced betrayal at some point or others from the relationships they considered and valued the most. However, the dejection and alienation experienced through such betrayal might have made it challenging for the participants to rekindle the lost trust in relationships, further impeding the development of social ties and the generation of hope considered essential for recovery and empowerment.

Mending Ties amidst Withering Hopes

Recalling Chapter 4, the life stories of Ayesha, Karunai, Shankar, Bijon, and Sujaya indicated how they started their uphill journey against the social sufferings towards recovery and empowerment to some extent. However, they lost momentum as they could not garner hope. While all these participants expressed contentment in their present situation, since they lacked hope, they did not find any meaning to continue their struggle to move beyond the status quo towards a potentially fulfilling direction in life. The absence of strong social ties and some not-so-strong connections threaded all these life stories together. It might help explain their inability to nurture hope, although they remained content with their present state.

Similar to the stories in Chapter 3, the lived experiences of the vignettes in Chapter 4 indicate a life of deprivation, dejection, and dehumanisation. After years of being oppressed by the patriarchal power processes, Ayesha, Karunai, Shankar, and Bijon *chose* to stay away from their families; however, Sujaya had no primary caregivers to take her back home.

Unlike the participants in Chapter 3, the vignettes in Chapter 4 developed some social ties with the mental health service community, particularly with their proxy caregivers. Sujaya and Karunai experienced developing some social ties within the mental health community, especially with their co-residents, based on mutual empathy and understanding. Rehabilitated into the community through the "Naya Daur" project of Iswar Sankalpa, Ayesha, and Bijon could bond with the community members of the neighbourhoods where they were staying. Even when engaged in menial jobs, both reported experiencing a reciprocal relationship of trust and respect with their employers. Their past experiences working in the unorganised sector might have been helpful for them in recreating such social networks.

Bijon, like Nalini, experienced a sense of comfort in leaving the uncertainties of the future at the mercy of the almighty. On the other hand, Shankar had created an intensely strong reciprocal bond with his proxy caregiver. Estranged by his family, Shankar experienced a purpose in life through this new meaningful bond. However, Ayesha, Karunai, Shankar, Bijon, and Sujaya found it challenging to extend their social bonds beyond a limited network. The absence of significant others and ageing and related physical ailments might have played a role in not maintaining their motivation to strengthen these ties further. While social ties are essential for community integration, the limited access of the mainstream community to the shelter residents might have interfered with an extension of the networks. On the other hand, Shankar, Bijon, and Ayesha could create networks in mainstream society beyond the mental health service community. However, none of the bonds they developed were meaningful enough to help them overcome the hurdles of social suffering towards a more hopeful future.

Developing Social Ties Tied with Hope

The life stories illustrated in Chapter 5 explored how some HMI persons, irrespective of their experiences of social suffering associated with downward mobilisation, could initiate and continue their journey back towards the mainstream. They had experienced exclusion and alienation at familial and social levels. Although they had experienced some meaningful and fulfilling relationships in their past, the death of their primary caregivers had rendered Chethana, Pushpavalli, and Damayanti homeless because other family members denied shouldering the caregiving responsibility. However, these participants could develop significant relationships successfully with the mental health community, including the service providers and their fellow residents at the shelter houses. As Tsai et al. (2012) identified, the mental health community could compensate for much *lost social support* and the limited social network. It could become a source of natural support for HMI individuals.

Some researchers (Abraham & Stein, 2009) caution against the service users' reliance on the mental health community. However, individuals with homelessness and SMI is one of the most socially alienated population, estranged from their primary and secondary care providers. For them, a meaningful social bond may provide a ray of hope for a meaningful future. Betrayed and alienated by their immediate social networks, the participants had reshaped and redefined their meaning of "home" and considered the shelter houses or their shared accommodation as their home (as noted at the beginning of this chapter). Consequently, the concept of family, which is integral to home for all of them, also got reshaped. The mental health community gave them the support and care they once expected from their familial relations. With mutual understanding and empathy, the mental health community thus became a place for them that could foster and rekindle those lost ties at familial and social levels. As a result, Chethana and Pushpavalli experienced a satisfying life as they lived in a shared house where there was independence, privacy, and reciprocity.

These participants also acknowledged the NGOs' vital role in making resources such as shelter, food, clothing, and medical facilities accessible. In

2016, for the first time, after two decades of advocacy, 102 women of The Banyan exercised their *right to vote* in the election that year, thereby overcoming the archaic Representation of the People Act, 1950, that disqualified a person who is "of unsound mind" to vote. The residents of The Banyan (Kumar, 2019) and Iswar Sankalpa also voted in the 2019 parliament election. Indeed, this remarkable change from being a taken-for-granted person living on the streets to being able to vote in elections could be possible because of the support they received from the NGOs.

Chethana and Pushpavalli further acknowledged how the NGOs facilitated their process of financial empowerment. While they experienced multiple hurdles in mainstream society to regain their footing following their diagnosis of mental illness (owing to the social stigma), the role of the NGOs was significantly important in helping them overcome this particular barrier. Similarly, providing them with the required *training to undertake a vocation of choice*, be it in baking or tailoring, or computer training appeared to be particularly beneficial.

The service providers further expedite the process of social networking and community integration for individuals with SMI. As identified by the participants, when introduced back to the mainstream community through the NGO, the chances of dejection were reduced significantly, mainly because the NGOs generally approached such employers who were accommodative. Damayanti highlighted this bridging role that the social worker played for her. It introduced her back to the mainstream community and strengthened their mutual bond further. Participants like Damayanti, Chethana, Pushpavalli, and Pradeepto talked about extending their social network beyond the mental health community to the mainstream community through workplace relations where they were accepted and entrusted with responsibilities.

While some developed new social ties replacing those that betrayed and estranged them, vignettes like Snigdha kept in them the hope of reuniting with their loved ones. She awaited to rekindle her relationship with her daughter. The hope of seeing her infant daughter once again and having a future with her kept Snigdha going (Padgett et al. 2008). In this next segment, I will discuss how the development of these new social ties helped rediscover valued social resources that helped in the upward mobilisation of HMI individuals.

Rediscovering the Valued Social Resources for Recovery and Empowerment

As Putnam (2000) posited, the Social Capital Theory focuses on positive reciprocal social ties, weak or strong, facilitating access to social resources (e.g., employment opportunity, financial support) that enable empowerment. The absence of such positive reciprocal social ties may hinder the accessibility to these social resources in the context of the vignettes, as observed in Chapter

3. The lack of meaningful and social relations might intensify the experience of social isolation, hindering the nurturance of hope and motivation and, in the long run, enabling recovery. Simultaneously, it may be difficult to envisage empowerment without these social resources.

Importantly, as noted by Pahwa et al. (2019) in their study, individuals with homelessness and SMI could gather (a) "*bonding social capital*," that is, "*resources obtained from close relationships*" (such as family relationships) besides (b) "*bridging social capital*," that is, "*resources* derived from acquaintances or *more professional relationships*, through ties to service providers, places of employment and people they met in cultural spaces" (p. 8, emphasis added). It appears that the participants mentioned in Chapter 4 initiated accessing "bridging social capital" without "bonding social capitals." However, ageing and related ailments, experiences of betrayal in the past, absence of meaningful past relationships or presence of significant others, and limited access to mainstream society apparently impeded being hopeful and motivated to access the social resources, that is, the potential *bridging social capital*. Thus, they shared their content with their status quo, that is, the availability of essential amenities through the NGOs, but could not perceive a potentially fulfilling future based on hope.

That developing social ties might facilitate access to social resources was apparent in the life stories of the vignettes presented in Chapter 5. As the *bridging social capital*, the mental health service community played a significant role in facilitating their access to social resources such as employment opportunities (including job hunting and training), besides helping overcome stigma at the workplace. Vignettes looking forward to employment also gathered their hope through the experiences of these fellow residents.

In the absence of significant others among familial relations, the vignettes could also extend their boundaries that were once limited to intimate groups that were developed through blood ties or intentional commitments like marriage. The socio-centric worldview (orientation of creating harmony within relationships) of the Indian society might have conditioned the participants in a more adaptive manner, where people, especially women, are trained since childhood to have the flexibility of broadening the circle of familial relations. While the concept, structure, and dynamics of family have been evolving in the neoliberal globalisation era among the "new middle class," "the essential characteristic of *conventional family value system is still existent*" (Patole, 2018, p. 23, emphasis added). Furthermore, as most of the vignettes belonged to a lower-middle SES that is more resistant to adopting modern lifestyles or values, the traditional collective values of the family system might have remained unaltered for them. Thus, they could conceptualise their fellow residents, service providers, or proxy caregivers as members of a "new family" after being dejected by and estranged from their family of origin or marriage. Participants, who shared a house or living arrangement where a family-like environment was mimicked in the "Home Again" project of The Banyan, expressed better satisfaction. The significance of these projects underlies their basic conceptualisation, where the "family-like environment" has been simulated, keeping in mind the notions of emotional security and commitment that family represents. In mimicking a "family-like environment," doing everyday chores, celebrating festivals, accompanying each other to the doctor, or welcoming guests, they committed to each other. This form of reciprocal commitment and concern based on mutual understanding and empathy, along with developing a robust social network, could also be observed in the vignettes, as presented in Chapter 5.

While betrayal experienced due to familial estrangement posed a barrier for many in developing social ties, family, particularly children, appeared to be the locus of all hope for those who had any. Their hope to rekindle their lost connections with their children became a critical source of support for the mothers.

While the valued social resources and their rediscovery through developing functional social ties helped the HMI individuals towards upward mobilisation, the resurrection of selfhood is the thrust that has initiated this process. In the following section, I would thus discuss how the resurrection of selfhood facilitated HMI individuals' experiences of recovery and empowerment.

Resurrecting Selfhood, Recovery, and Empowerment

Life-long struggle and social suffering due to adverse interpersonal, institutional, or structural conditions may threaten the coherence of meanings one associates with one's selfhood ("Who am I?"). Cassell (2004) illustrated the relationship one has with oneself as "self," and "self-esteem, self-approval, self-love (and their opposites) are emotional expressions of the relationship of a self to itself." (p. 39). The suffering experienced by the participants "from what they have lost of themselves concerning the world of objects, events, and relationships" (Cassell, 2004) threatened the intactness, coherence, and integrity of this relationship. Consequently, it threatened self-esteem, self-value, and self-love.

Classically, SMI was considered a "distortion of self" (e.g., Freud, 1910; Fromm-Reichmann, 1950, as cited in Davidson & Strauss, 1992). While it holds little or no value as a diagnostic characteristic today, phenomenologically, "sense of self continues to provide a key theoretical construct in the understanding and treatment of these disorders" (Davidson & Strauss, 1992, p. 132), particularly in the recovery-based model of mental health service. Also, the stigmatised identities of "homeless" and "mentally ill" might negatively affect the concept of self, as most participants talked about losing self-esteem or self-confidence at some point. Deegan (1996) reflected on her experience of suffering from schizophrenia, which resonated with many of the vignettes.

> Giving up was not a problem; it was a solution. It was a solution because it protected me from wanting anything. If I didn't want anything, then it couldn't be taken away. If I didn't try, then I wouldn't

have to undergo another failure. If I didn't care, then nothing could hurt me again. My heart became hardened.

(p. 93)

The recovery-based model of mental health has thus placed the resurrection of the notions of selfhood at its core. Roberts and Wolfson (2004) reflected that the process of recovery in SMI begins with "regaining a sense of self, of taking control and responsibility, often combining optimism for the future with acceptance of the past" (p. 40). The categories of "meaning of living a satisfactory life" and "meaning of living a contributing life" in the context of the vignettes who experienced them have evolved around the resurrection of selfhood.

Though recovery and empowerment have appeared to be complementary for a marginalised population like the HMI individuals, despite its integral role in recovery, notions of selfhood remained relatively unexplored in the context of empowerment. While the literature has posited *recovery* as a *personal* process, *empowerment* has been conceptualised as a *collective community-involved* process (Zimmerman, 2000). However, the participants in my study who shared experiences of being empowered highlighted the importance of "resurrecting selfhood," that is, "feeling the need for self-sufficiency and self-sustenance as an indispensable aspect of empowering oneself." The empowerment process also begins with the rediscovery of selfhood. It continues as the vignettes address their "self-empowerment" need to be "self-dependent," ensuring a secure and stable future for "self and significant others" (where they would not be considered dispensable for not being financially empowered), and taking up or planning social or income-generation activities passionately to provide "self" with a sense of empowerment.

Being empowered was identified by the vignettes as restoring their pride and dignity with the help of some critical enablers like "regaining functional prowess," both physical and cognitive, and developing new purpose and meaning in life. In addition, all the vignettes with experiences of empowerment reflected the benefit of being employed, having financial security, particularly for their old age, giving back to society, earning respect in return, and thereby living a "contributing" life. This was also evident in the findings of Pahwa et al. (2019), where an empowered individual would show an array of positive outcomes, both physically and emotionally. The literature has further documented additional benefits that the vignettes experienced, including social and emotional well-being and improved overall quality of life.

Implications

This book highlights some theoretical-methodological and applied-policy implications that help academicians, clinicians, policymakers, and other stakeholders have a more nuanced understanding of the HMI populations and provide them with services that might help to serve them more holistically beyond clinical recovery.

Theoretical and Methodological Implications

Social Suffering, Recovery, and Empowerment: Intersectionality-Focused Frameworks: This book explores how the "dual burden" of being *homeless* and *mentally ill* influences these individuals; the downward social drift and increased risk of impoverishment, being denied their "identity" and dignity in the process. The entire spectrum of this book, from losing their homes to debilitating mental health conditions, the process of recovery, and the challenges faced, provides a bird's eye view of the struggles of the HMI population. These also point to various interventions that could have been possible (and are needed) at various stages of their life journey.

Contextualising Recovery and Empowerment: Research in the last three decades has consistently indicated a close association between homelessness and mental illness (Bhugra, 2007; Patel & Kleinman, 2003; Susser et al., 1990). Authors have recommended exploring the role of recovery and hope as factors that might provide for psychiatric rehabilitation in HMI (Bhugra, 2007; Gopikumar et al., 2015; Moorkath et al., 2018). Yet, little research has been done to understand the factors or self and context-related processes that might accelerate their upward mobilisation. This was an attempt to explore and contextualise the lived experiences of the HMI individuals in the Indian setup (that emphasises a socio-centric worldview about selfhood and relationships) through recovery and empowerment.

Listening to the Unheard through Humanising Ethnographic Space: The possibility of including their context and voices has hardly been focused on in prior studies despite the call for ethnographic studies. By co-constructing meanings with the participants about the activities that they resort to survive exorbitantly adverse situations, this study tends to get closer to their context of life and voice. Listening to their lived experiences (and *silences*) of social suffering within the hierarchical power processes, engaging with their narratives compassionately, and presenting the insights to the potential stakeholders have been an attempt in this study towards humanising their existence (Sampson, 1993). Their lived experiences and voices tell us explicitly in their *own words* about their difficulties, marginalisation and their "unmet needs." Especially in a country that houses a significant number of the world's homeless population, the narratives of the participants might help to identify them through their "lost identity" and humanise their sufferings.

Beyond Therapeutic Nihilism: Towards Mental Healthcare in Relational Context: Their training based on the medical model often does not encourage mental healthcare professionals to look beyond symptoms and placement for the HMI individuals. In the absence of restitution, when families are not found, the generally observed therapeutic nihilism of biomedically trained service providers in the Indian setting might create a vacuum as far as meaningful community-based rehabilitation is concerned. Thus, for meaningful rehabilitation efforts for HMI persons, this book highlights and re-emphasised the need to use a more realistic *critical*, *contextual* paradigm to identify them as "human beings" (rather than "patients") who live their lives within relational contexts – equitable-and-caring or hierarchical-and-exclusionary.

Applied and Policy-Related Implications

Need to Integrate Mental Health into Primary Healthcare: It is already established that India has been facing an exponentially increasing treatment gap in the field of mental health. With a population of over a billion in India, the National Mental Health Survey (NMHS), in 2016, data revealed a huge "mental health gap" of 85.4% and one in five individuals suffering from a mental health disorder. There are 0.75 psychiatrists/1,00,000 Indian population compared to 6/1,00,000 in high-income countries (Garg et al., 2019). The NMHS also showed a disproportionate distribution of services, with most resources clustered in urban cities, creating a huge gap in rural India. And this *treatment gap* resonated through all the life stories collected during my fieldwork. While one cannot readily bridge such a vast gap, some attempts may surely be made towards that direction. As the life stories indicated, many participants experienced the suffering associated with SMI (including homelessness) primarily because early diagnosis and treatment were absent. Even when they were taken to the general physicians during a prodromal phase (e.g., Damayanti), the diagnosis was not made.

Furthermore, inadequate knowledge and associated apathy among the general physicians only worsened their suffering (e.g., Sujaya). This brings us back to the discussion about whether mental health must become an integral part of the primary healthcare system. As witnessed through the life stories, the burden of mental illness is enormous, both on the highly vulnerable end-users such as HMI persons and on caregivers. A lot of the associated suffering may be minimised if the individual receives treatment adequately and timely. Integrating mental health treatment in primary healthcare facilities would not only make treatment accessible to the end-users, particularly in rural India but would also make it affordable and cost-effective (Collins et al., 2011; Funk et al., 2008).

Need for Community-Based Intervention: Naya Daur, the community-based intervention programme that the NGO Iswar Sankalpa has been running for the past decade in Kolkata, presents an excellent example of how a medico-social issue like homelessness-SMI can be addressed (at least locally) with a collaborative integration among mental health professionals, social workers, and community. In this case, the Kolkata Municipal Corporation's proactive participation helped the NGO run the intervention successfully across the city. Naya Daur, as the service providers of Iswar Sankalpa, highlighted, not only helped them in reaching out to more service users than they could otherwise help within the restricted resources of shelter houses but also helped them in increasing awareness and dealing with the stigma about mental health within the community. The proxy caregivers that they created as part of this intervention are community members with no background in mental health treatment. Their sensibility and humanity are the most substantial resource that the NGO has utilised and allocated effectively. While it is true that not every community might react in the same way to this model of intervention as Kolkata did (a lot would depend on the socio-cultural context of the city), however, by understanding the need and temperament of specific communities, tailor-made interventions might be planned to bridge the treatment gap highly vulnerable groups such as HMI persons further.

Need to Move beyond Clinical Recovery: The life stories have also reaffirmed the need to move beyond the "impairment only" understanding of the HMI population. As the study has indicated, neither homelessness nor SMI should mark the end of the journey of progressive, satisfying or contributory life for them. With adequate clinical as well as community-based rehabilitation premised on the availability of valued social or relational resources, they generally have all the potential for upward mobilisation. The interventions thus need to include help for the individuals, particularly in identifying their voices and rediscovering the valued social resources that might aid them in their journey towards recovery and empowerment.

Nurturing "Hope" to Enable Recovery and Empowerment: The insights developed from the life stories of the participants have helped in understanding that "hope" as a way of life has made a marked difference in the HMI individuals' journeys towards recovery and empowerment. While hope has helped them in mending broken social ties and developing new ties, the absence of it restricted the individuals from taking the initiative to rejuvenate their social support and thereby keeping within bounds their accessibility to valued social resources. The intervention and rehabilitation processes, thus, might need to address and *harness an individual's social connections* through which further resources might be generated to help them move towards recovery and empowerment. Identifying the various mechanisms that the individuals have been employing to form social ties (e.g., interaction with community members or fellow co-residents) might help in developing more meaningful services. The communication and interaction that one has with their co-residents are often dependent on mutual understanding and empathy. Identifying such relationships and nurturing them might become potential sources of strength and positive social ties. Furthermore, healing the estranged relationships with families or reconnecting dormant ties (e.g., Damayanti with her old student, Muraad with his old classmate) might help them in the process of not only developing the social ties but would also bridge the gap in their connectedness that they might experience due to the social alienation process.

Identifying Gaps in Services: This book might help the service providers to have an insight into the gaps in their services, identify their resources and also the personal resources of the HMI individuals that can enhance service provision. The fact that both the service providers and service users identified some of the common challenges that they experience (e.g., intra-institutional hierarchies) might help them in taking effective measures to tackle the issue. Furthermore, as many residents highlighted the struggles associated with living in the shelter houses once they got clinically recovered, the NGOs need to address such struggles towards a more meaningful rehabilitation. However, the unavailability of an adequate budget often makes it difficult for the service providers to execute the plans that might help in facilitating recovery and empowerment. Proactive participation of policymakers and other stakeholders might help to meet the structural and systemic challenges experienced by the service providers. With a 85.4% treatment gap, while the vast responsibility lies with the NGO sector to bridge this gap (Patel & Thara, 2003), the poor resource allocation and apathy of stakeholders often make it an unsurmountable struggle for them, especially when it comes to serving those who have mental illness and are homeless at the same time due to social suffering and stigma. The social support or community rehabilitation model might help the NGOs to deal with the lack of human resource capacity that they experience because of the transient nature of the HMI population. Volunteers, social workers, and community members might be trained to follow up with identified homeless persons on the streets and develop a liaison with legal and administrative services so that if they move from the particular community, they could be tracked down and provided with the required services (food, medicine, etc.)

Policy and Legislations: Even after revising the previous act after three decades, the Mental Healthcare Act of 2017 has not adequately addressed the issue of HMI individuals or similarly vulnerable populations owing to its inherent focus on clinical recovery. Also, the inadequate budget allocation for rehabilitation camps and shelter homes for the homeless forces them to shut down or become ineffective. The service providers identified that rehabilitation into the community often become challenging due to the inadequacy of fund that might help them to rent houses for shared-home purposes for recovered individuals. The Ministry of Micro, Small and Medium Enterprises needs to promote the vocational units of the various NGOs that are working towards ensuring the financial and social empowerment of the HMI individuals. Furthermore, there is no scope for adequate legal remedy for abuse of mentally ill individuals by family members following restitution or for non-reporting their leaving home. Like the Indian Penal Code has made provision for mandatory reporting of child abuse under the Prevention of Child Sexual Offence, legislative provisions should be made that might help this extremely vulnerable population from further abuses.

Future Directions

Longitudinal follow-up studies with an action research orientation to explore the spectrum of homelessness (from being homeless to social recovery/rehabilitation) and implement the *implications of the findings* of this study presented above need to be taken up. It is crucial to explore the perspectives of the family members of HMI persons for the prevention of poorer mental health as well as the socio-economic conditions of the HMI persons. Furthermore, studies of mental health on various *vulnerable groups within the homeless* (children, adolescents, physically or intellectually disabled) need to be taken up. Finally, the post-COVID-19 situation demands that an urgent exploration of their continued struggle during the pandemic needs to be done towards interventions for their protection and safety.

Note

1 According to Rosen et al. (2006), prodromal phase is "the period of subclinical signs and symptoms that precedes the onset of psychosis is referred to as the prodrome. The prodromal period can last from weeks to several years, and comorbid disorders are very common during this period." Initiating treatment and providing adequate social and emotional support may be significant in prevention.

References

Abraham, K. M., & Stein, C. H. (2009). Case managers' expectations about employment for people with psychiatric disabilities. *Psychiatric Rehabilitation Journal, 33*(1), 9.

Adichie, C. N. (2014). *We should all be feminists*. Vintage.

Anthony, W. A. (1993). Recovery from mental illness: The guiding vision of the Mental Health Service System in the 1990s. *Psychosocial Rehabilitation Journal, 16*(4), 11.

Anthony, W. A., Cohen, M. R., Farkas, M. D., & Gagne, C. (2002). *Psychiatric rehabilitation: Center for psychiatric rehabilitation*. Boston, MA: Sargent College of Health and Rehabilitation Sciences Boston University.

Bhatia, S., & Priya, K. R. (2018). Decolonising culture: Euro-American psychology and the shaping of neoliberal selves in India. *Theory & Psychology, 28*(5), 645–668. https://doi.org/10.1177/0959354318791315

Bhugra, D. (Ed.). (2007). *Homelessness and mental health*. Cambridge University Press.

Carstensen, L. L., Isaacowitz, D. M., & Charles, S. T. (1999). Taking time seriously: A theory of socioemotional selectivity. *American Psychologist, 54*(3), 165.

Cassell, E. J. (2004). *The nature of suffering and the goals of medicine* (2nd ed.). Oxford.

Charmaz, K. (2002). Stories and silences: Disclosures and self in chronic illness. *Qualitative inquiry, 8*(3), 302–328.

Charmaz, K. (2020). Experiencing stigma and exclusion: The influence of neoliberal perspectives, practices, and policies on living with chronic illness and disability. *Symbolic Interaction, 43*(1), 21–45.

Collins, P. Y., Patel, V., Joestl, S. S., March, D., Insel, T. R., Daar, A. S., Bordin, I. A., Costello, E. J., Durkin, M., Fairburn, C., Glass, R. I., Hall, W., Huang, Y., Hyman, S. E., Jamison, K., Kaaya, S., Kapur, S., Kleinman, A., Ogunniyi, A., ... Walport, M. (2011). Grand challenges in global mental health. *Nature, 475*(7354), 27–30.

Corrigan, P. W., Mueser, K. T., Bond, G. R., Drake, R. E., & Solomon, P. (2008). *Principles and practice of psychiatric rehabilitation: An empirical approach.* Guilford Press.

Crime in India – 2018 Statistics Volume 1. (2020). Retrieved July 10, 2020, from https://ncrb.gov.in/en/crime-india-2018

Davidson, L., & Strauss, J. S. (1992). Sense of self in recovery from severe mental illness. *British Journal of Medical Psychology, 65*(2), 131–145.

Deegan, P. (1996). Recovery as a journey of the heart. *Psychiatric Rehabilitation Journal, 19*(3), 91.

Funk, M., Saraceno, B., Drew, N., & Faydi, E. (2008). Integrating mental health into primary healthcare. *Mental Health in Family Medicine, 5*(1), 5–8.

Garg, K., Kumar, C. N., & Chandra, P. S. (2019). Number of psychiatrists in India: Baby steps forward, but a long way to go. *Indian Journal of Psychiatry, 61*(1), 104–105. https://doi.org/10.4103/psychiatry.IndianJPsychiatry_7_18

Geetha, V. (2002). *Gender (Theorizing feminism).* Stree.

Goldberg, S. (1979). *Male dominance: The inevitability of patriarchy.* Sphere.

Gopikumar, V., Easwaran, K., Ravi, M., Jude, N., & Bunders, J. (2015). Mimicking family like attributes to enable a state of personal recovery for persons with mental illness in Institutional Care Settings. *International Journal of Mental Health Systems, 9*(1), 30.

How will the homeless citizens get Aadhaar? Sc asks Government (2018, January 10). *Anandabazar Patrika.* Retrieved from https://www.anandabazar.com/national/how-will-the-homeless-citizens-get-aadhaar-sc-asks-government-dgtl-1.738038?ref=stry dtl-rltd-national, http://www.un.org/documents/ga/res/48/a48r104.htm

Hunnicutt, G. (2009). Varieties of patriarchy and violence against women: Resurrecting "Patriarchy" as a theoretical tool. *Violence against Women, 15*(5), 553–573.

Khalifeh, H., & Dean, K. (2010). Gender and violence against people with severe mental illness. *International Review of Psychiatry, 22*(5), 535–546.

Kleinman, A., Das, V., Lock, M., & Lock, M. M. (Eds.). (1997). *Social suffering.* University of California Press.

Krishnaraj, M. (2017). [Foreword]. In J. Bagchi (Author), *Interrogating motherhood (Theorizing Feminism)* [eBook Edition]. Sage.

Kumar, A., Nizamie, S. H., & Srivastava, N. K. (2013). Violence against women and mental health. *Mental Health & Prevention, 1*(1), 4–10.

Kumar, K. (2019, March 28). Franchise is the voice that people with mental illness need: Chennai news. *Times of India.* Retrieved August 10, 2020, from https://timesofindia.indiatimes.com/city/chennai/franchise-is-the-voice-that-people-with-mental-illness-need/articleshow/68605364.cms

Lang, R. (2000). The role of NGOs in the process of empowerment and social trans-formation of people with disabilities. *Asia Pacific Disability Rehabilitation Journal, 1*(1), 1–19.

Lund, C. (2014). Poverty and mental health: Towards a research agenda for low and middle-income countries. Commentary on Tampubolon and Hanandita (2014). *Social Science & Medicine, 111,* 134e136.

Mills, C. (2018). From 'Invisible Problem' to global priority: The inclusion of mental health in the sustainable development goals. *Development and Change*, *49*(3), 843–866. https://doi.org/10.1111/dech.12397

Moorkath, F., Vranda, M. N., & Naveenkumar, C. (2018). Lives without roots: Institutionalized homeless women with Chronic Mental Illness. *Indian Journal of Psychological Medicine*, *40*(5), 476.

National Crime Records Bureau. (2021). Retrieved December 11, 2022, from https://ncrb.gov.in/en/Crime-in-India-2021

Padgett, D. K., Henwood, B., Abrams, C., & Drake, R. E. (2008). Social relationships among persons who have experienced serious mental illness, substance abuse, and homelessness: Implications for recovery. *American Journal of Orthopsychiatry*, *78*(3), 333–339.

Pahwa, R., Smith, M. E., Yuan, Y., & Padgett, D. (2019). The ties that bind and unbound ties: Experiences of formerly homeless individuals in recovery from serious mental illness and substance use. *Qualitative Health Research*, *29*(9), 1313–1323.

Patel, V., & Kleinman, A. (2003). Poverty and common mental disorders in developing countries. *Bulletin of the World Health Organization*, *81*(8), 609–615.

Patel, V., & Thara, R. (2003). Introduction: The role of NGOs in mental health care. In V. Patel & R. Thara (Eds.), *Meeting the mental health needs of developing countries: NGO innovations in India* (pp. 1–19). Sage Publications India.

Patole, J. (2018). The impact of globalization on the new middle class family in India. *IOSR Journal of Humanities and Social Science*, *23*(1), 6–14.

Putnam, R. D. (2000). *Bowling alone: The collapse and revival of American community*. Simon & Schuster.

Read, J. (2010). Can poverty drive you mad? 'Schizophrenia', socio-economic status and the case for primary prevention. *New Zealand Journal of Psychology*, *39*(2), 7–19.

Roberts, G., & Wolfson, P. (2004). The rediscovery of recovery: Open to all. *Advances in Psychiatric Treatment*, *10*(1), 37–48.

Rosen, J. L., Miller, T. J., D'Andrea, J. T., McGlashan, T. H., & Woods, S. W. (2006). Comorbid diagnoses in patients meeting criteria for the schizophrenia prodrome. *Schizophrenia Research*, *85*(1–3), 124–131.

Sahoo, D. M. (2014). An analysis of widowhood in India: A global perspective. *International Journal of Multidisciplinary and Current Research*, *2*(3), 45–58.

Sampson, E. E. (1993). Identity politics: Challenges to psychology's understanding. *American Psychologist*, *48*(12), 1219.

Sharma, D. & Priya, K. R. (2020, March 28). Excluded in rehabilitation: Disability in the neo-liberal Era? *Economic and Political Weekly*, *55*(13), 12–15.

Shibusawa, T., & Padgett, D. (2009). The experiences of "Aging" among formerly homeless adults with Chronic Mental Illness: A qualitative study. *Journal of Aging Studies*, *23*(3), 188–196.

Susmitha, B. (2016). Domestic violence: Causes, impact and remedial measures. *Social Change*, *46*(4), 602–610.

Susser, E., Goldfinger, S. M., & White, A. (1990). Some clinical approaches to the homeless mentally ill. *Community Mental Health Journal*, *26*(5), 463–480.

Tipple, A. G., & Speak, S. E. (2005). *Homelessness in developing countries*. Newcastle upon Tyne, Global Urban Research Unit, University of Newcastle upon Tyne.

Tsai, J., Rosenheck, R. A., & McGuire, J. F. (2012). Comparison of outcomes of homeless female and male veterans in transitional housing. *Community Mental Health Journal, 48*(6), 705–710.

United Nations. (1993). *Declaration on the elimination of violence against women.* Geneva, Switzerland: United Nations.

Walby, S. (1990). *Theorizing patriarchy.* Basil Blackwell.

Zimmerman, M. A. (2000). Empowerment theory. In J. Rappaport & E. Seidman (Eds.), *Handbook of community psychology* (pp. 43–63). Springer Science & Business Media.

Appendix I
Life Story Interview Guide for Service Users

Each interview begins with the following question:

Tell me how you came to this point.

This question is likely to help to put the participants at ease and establish rapport before delving into more sensitive issues.

1. What do you remember about your childhood?
2. As you were growing up, who do you think in your family and friends had the most significant positive role in your life and how? (emotional, motivational)
3. As you were growing up, who do you think in your family and friends had the most significant negative role in your life and how? How did you deal with that? (emotional, motivational)
4. What do you remember as the beginning of these problems? (precipitating factors)
5. What do you think of your illness?
6. What is the experience of developing this illness?
7. How did you feel when you were first diagnosed? (emotional, cognitive, behavioural)
8. How do you think your life has been affected by your illness? (personal, interpersonal, social, functional)
9. Has there been no illness, how do you think your life would have been different? (personal, interpersonal, social, functional)
10. How do these changes make you feel? (emotional, cognitive, behavioural)
11. What has been your experience of living with it so far?
12. What do you think of other people's reactions to this? (family members, fellow residents, service providers)
13. What is the meaning of home? (beyond four walls with a roof)
14. What is homelessness to you?
15. What do you consider yourself now, and why? (with or without a home)
16. Describe a situation where you were in danger, and how did you know this?
17. What behaviours do you think put you at risk?

18. What did you do to avoid dangerous situations?
19. What factors made it hard for you to avoid unsafe situations?
20. Describe what you consider a safe area?
21. What would you tell someone living on the streets to do to avoid harm?
22. What is your meaning of hope?
23. What are the sources from which you gain your hope? (personal, relational, social, situational)
24. What do you hope for?
25. What are your needs? What do you think of them? (adequately met or not)
26. What do you think of your future? (personal, interpersonal, social, occupational)
27. What are the ways you think you can help yourself to settle down independently beyond this shelter house?
28. How do you think you are helping others to live their life?
29. How do you think you can help others to live their life?
30. Ten years later... Where do you see yourself? (personal, interpersonal, social, occupational)
31. What do you dream of doing in the future? How do you think you can do that?
32. What are the strengths that have helped you till date to fight this journey?
33. What has been helpful/encouraging in dealing with your problems?
34. How have you coped with these problems of homelessness and mental illness together?
35. What are the services that the service providers provide you with?
36. What aspects of these services do you find helpful to build up an independent life outside these premises?
37. What aspects of the services do you find unhelpful to build up an independent life outside these premises?
38. What more do you think you need?

Appendix II
Semi-Structured Interview for Service Providers

1. What is the service users' (the homeless individuals diagnosed with severe mental illnesses) meaning of hope?
2. What are the sources from which service users gain their hope? (personal, relational, social, situational)
3. What do service users hope for?
4. What are service users' needs? (adequately met or not)
5. What are the ways you think service users can help themselves to settle down independently beyond this shelter house?
6. How do you think service users are helping others to live their life?
7. How do you think service users can help others to live their life?
8. What do service users generally think of doing in the future? (personal, interpersonal, social, occupational). How do you think they can do that?
9. What do you think are service users' strengths that have helped them till date to fight this journey?
10. What do you think have been helpful/encouraging in dealing with their service users' problems?
11. How do you think service users have coped with these problems of homelessness and mental illness together?
12. What are the services that you provide the service users with?
13. What aspects of these services do you find helpful to build up an independent life outside these premises for service users?
14. What aspects of the services do you find unhelpful to build up an independent life outside these premises for service users?
15. What more do you think service users' need?
16. What are your experiences of working with this population?
17. What effect does your service have on the service users?
18. What effect does your work have on your relationship with the service users?
19. What motivates you to keep on doing this work?
20. What are the different challenges that you face in the process of providing service to this population? (personal, interpersonal, systemic, structural, social, economic)

Appendix III
Operational Definitions of Categories

Category	Subcategory	Definition
Experience of Social Suffering Associated with the Downward Mobilisation in HMI Persons (Figure 2.1)	Exclusion and Victimisation Due to Patriarchal Power Processes	Experiencing dehumanisation on being subjected to oppression and exploitation by patriarchal power processes
	Meaning of Home and Homelessness	Perceiving home as a space that may provide independent agency to access resources, where one is settled and rooted with loved ones and is being mutually cared for. On the contrary, homelessness is perceived as being uprooted, without happiness, peace, and comfort in the company of loved ones.
	The Lived Experiences of Homelessness	Suffering associated with experiencing homelessness: Feeling dehumanised and humiliated on being physically, sexually, or emotionally tormented due to being vulnerable as a homeless. Surviving homelessness: Being forced to learn strategies (like identifying safe zones and food providers) to survive homelessness.
	The Lived Experiences of Surviving SMI	• Meaning making of symptoms and suffering associated with SMI • Double Jeopardy of being unaware of and apathetic nature of service provision • Consequences of SMI: Experiencing dehumanisation and deprivation due to the brunt of SMI through the associated multifaceted losses (personal/interpersonal/socioeconomic) and stigma.
Challenges to the Process of Recovery and Empowerment (Figure 2.2)	Inaccessibility to Resources Related to Socioeconomic and Community-based Constraints	Experiencing overwhelming helplessness due to inaccessibility to resources due to the absence of adequate social support and financial security impedes recovery and empowerment
	Inaccessibility to Resources Related to Motivational Constraints:	Feeling of overwhelming hopelessness because of (a) inaccessibility to resources due to the lack of control over treatment-resistant symptoms and (b) difficulty relating to the mainstream society that impedes the process of recovery and empowerment towards a realistic future.
	Consequences of Being Dependent on the NGO:	Experience of being humiliated, unheard, and uncared for due to lack of space for one's voice and independence within the hierarchical system of the NGO.

Process of Recovery and Empowerment (Figure 2.3)	Role of NGO and Community in Providing Resources and Unconditional Acceptance	The sense of developing and maintaining meaning and purpose in life is facilitated by the NGOs and community by being provided with resources and unconditional acceptance.
	Meaning of Living a Satisfactory Life	**Contentment with current status:** Experiencing satisfaction and contentment in the present way of life where one perceives oneself as having a relatively better quality of life compared to past experiences of extreme suffering at familial and societal levels, along with the resourcelessness of homelessness and symptoms of SMI.
		Regaining functional prowess: Experiencing meaning and satisfaction in life by regaining functional abilities (both physical and cognitive) that have been compromised due to repercussions of suffering homelessness and chronic SMI.
		Developing new purpose and meaning in life
		Hopes for a better future: Meaning of hope embedded in the meaning of the future where (a) self is perceived as independent, self-sufficient, fulfilling the dreams that have previously been denied, and (b) the essential requirement of being physically and mentally healthy is fulfilled
		Sources of hope and strength: The sources of hope and strength embedded in self, significant others, or God or having no other alternative but to survive
	Meaning of Living a Contributing Life	**Re-developing social support and social network:** Experiencing a purpose in life by creating social support and social network through (a)re-kindling lost trust in significant others and (b)developing new meaningful relationships based on empathy and mutual understanding.
		Significant impact on others: Experiencing self-satisfaction, meaning, and purpose of existence on having a substantial impact on and contribution to others' lives by being resourceful.
	Relationship Between the Notions of Selfhood and Self-Empowerment	**Resurrecting selfhood:** Feeling the need for self-sufficiency and self-sustenance as an indispensable aspect of empowering oneself.
		Addressing self-empowerment needs: Experiencing the necessity to empower oneself to be self-dependent, ensuring a secure and stable future for the self and children, where s/he would not be considered dispensable for not being financially empowered.
		Empowerment endeavours: Undertaking or planning endeavours passionately to provide oneself with an empowered status (financially and socially self-sufficient) with the help of NGO/community and past experiences of empowerment (previous job or business experiences.

(Continued)

Category	Subcategory	Definition
Experience of Service Providers in Facilitating the Process of Recovery and Empowerment in HMI Persons	**Challenges in Providing Service**	Experiencing extensive difficulty in providing service due to a) lack of existing resources and support at a systemic level, b) lack of awareness about mental illness among various stakeholders (government officials, primary health-care system) and c) intra-institutional hierarchy.
	Motivational Processes	Intrinsic motivation (also induced by personal losses) of serving the extremely marginalised population getting reinforcement of witnessing the process of recovery and empowerment among HMI persons.

Index

For Product Safety Concerns and Information please contact our EU
representative GPSR@taylorandfrancis.com
Taylor & Francis Verlag GmbH, Kaufingerstraße 24, 80331 München, Germany